PAY FOR
YOUR GRADUATE
NURSING EDUCATION
WITHOUT
GOING BROKE

Carl Buck, MS, CCPS, is a college financial aid expert with more than 30 years of experience guiding students, parents, and educators on matters related to how to pay for college.

As the former director of financial aid at leading institutions such as Rice University and Rutgers University and director of financial aid counseling at the University of California, Los Angeles (UCLA), Carl brings his insight and unique "inside" perspective to families challenged with keeping up with the rising cost of college for both undergraduate and graduate students.

Carl's prior publication *Get a Jump! The Student Aid Answer Book* was distributed to thousands of high schools across the country.

Carl has appeared on numerous talk shows and has been extensively quoted on college financial aid matters in leading media, such as *The New York Times, The Wall Street Journal, Kiplinger's Personal Finance,* and Bloomberg Radio. Most recently, Carl served as a vice president, Chase Student Loans, and a senior consultant, Discover Student Loans.

Carl earned both his bachelor's and master's degrees from Emerson College.

Rick Darvis, CPA, CCPS, is recognized as one of the leading experts in the financial planning field. He has written several books, developed financial software, and trained financial professionals across the United States. His knowledge has enabled him to be invited to speak on financial and business development topics to his contemporaries at state Certified Public Accountant (CPA) and Financial Planning Association (FPA) conferences in more than 40 states. He has been a featured speaker at the FPA's Success Forum, the Northeast/Mid-Atlantic National Association of Personal Financial Advisors (NAPFA) regional conference, the National Employee Benefit Forum, the New York State Society of CPAs Personal Financial Planning Conference, and the AICPA Conference on Tax Strategies for the High-Income Individual. Rick has also given seminars for the University of Arizona and the New York State Financial Aid Administrators Association.

Rick's accomplishments in the financial planning field are:

- Coauthor of *Paying for College: Tax Strategies and Financial Aid,* a guide published by the American Institute of CPAs on college planning for accountants and financial advisers
- Contributing author of the guidebook *Personal Financial Planning*
- Coauthor of *Planning for College Costs,* a guidebook on college financial planning for accountants and financial advisers
- Author of *A Roadmap to College & Retirement—Without Going Broke,* a book designed to link college planning to retirement planning
- Quoted in *Forbes,* CNNfn, *Newsweek, U.S. News and World Report, Money, Business Week, Kiplinger's Personal Finance, The New York Times, SmartMoney, The Wall Street Journal, Bloomberg Personal Finance,* Bankrate, *The Nation's Business, Financial Advisor,* Dow Jones Newswires, On Investing, Knight Ridder News, Mutual Fund Market News, *Research, Practical Accountant, Offspring, LIMRA's Market Facts, NAPFA Advisor,* and *AICPA's Planner*

PAY FOR YOUR GRADUATE NURSING EDUCATION WITHOUT GOING BROKE

Tips From the Pros

Carl Buck, MS, CCPS

Rick Darvis, CPA, CCPS

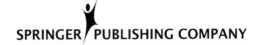

SPRINGER PUBLISHING COMPANY

Springer Publishing Company, LLC
11 West 42nd Street
New York, NY 10036
www.springerpub.com
http://connect.springerpub.com

Acquisitions Editor: Elizabeth Nieginski
Compositor: Amnet Systems

ISBN: 978-0-8261-4212-2
ebook ISBN: 978-0-8261-4227-6
DOI:10.1891/9780826142276

20 21 22 23 24/ 5 4 3 2 1

The author and the publisher of this Work have made every effort to use sources believed to be reliable to provide information that is accurate and compatible with the standards generally accepted at the time of publication. The author and publisher shall not be liable for any special, consequential, or exemplary damages resulting, in whole or in part, from the readers' use of, or reliance on, the information contained in this book. The publisher has no responsibility for the persistence or accuracy of URLs for external or third-party Internet websites referred to in this publication and does not guarantee that any content on such websites is, or will remain, accurate or appropriate.

Library of Congress Cataloging-in-Publication Data

Names: Buck, Carl, author. | Darvis, Rick, author.
Title: Pay for your graduate nursing education without going broke :
   tips from the pros / Carl Buck, Rick Darvis.
Description: New York, NY : Springer Publishing Company, [2020] | Includes
   bibliographical references and index.
Identifiers: LCCN 2019046722 (print) | LCCN 2019046723 (ebook) |
   ISBN 9780826142122 (paperback) | ISBN 9780826142276 (ebook)
Subjects: MESH: Education, Nursing, Graduate—economics | Financial Support |
   United States
Classification: LCC RT75 (print) | LCC RT75 (ebook) | NLM WY 18.5 |
   DDC 610.73071/1—dc23
LC record available at https://lccn.loc.gov/2019046722
LC ebook record available at https://lccn.loc.gov/2019046723

Contact us to receive discount rates on bulk purchases.
We can also customize our books to meet your needs.
For more information please contact: sales@springerpub.com

Publisher's Note: New and used products purchased from third-party sellers are not guaranteed for quality, authenticity, or access to any included digital components.

Printed in the United States of America.

CONTENTS

CONTRIBUTOR

John Schofield is a consultant to the National Institute of Certified College Planners and to College Funding Inc. These national organizations provide college planning education and support to families and financial professionals. John has firsthand experience with the challenges of obtaining an education in the medical profession.

PREFACE

"It's a gigantic mess." So spoke a well-respected professor of nursing when discussing the graduate nursing college financing landscape—and we agree.

Understanding the undergraduate college financial aid application process is daunting enough, but entering the unknown nuances of graduate nursing financial aid encompassing need- and merit-based grants, scholarships, stipends, "tuition free" work requirements, loan options, loan repayments, and loan forgiveness can be overwhelming.

Well, the good news is that this book offers constructive guidance, substantive information on financial strategies, and strategies on how to let Uncle Sam not only support your grad college costs with free money but also assist with utilizing tax initiatives for help with mortgages and retirement.

We tried to take into account that there are many profiles of a graduate nursing student: a single student in his or her twenties going from undergrad to MSN, or a nurse who decides to return to grad school after working a few years, or a nurse who has a family with kids in college or who are about to enter college. Regardless of your profile, we have provided case studies that you can identify with and consider real-life funding solutions. Life is meant to be enjoyed, not endured!

We offer advice on how, when, and why to appeal a grad nursing financial aid offer—and how to interact and develop a "partnership" with the financial aid office.

Obtaining grad nursing funding availability and understanding the processes involved is at times like walking into a hornet's nest. For example, did you know that some nursing grad schools want to know your parent's income when submitting the Free Application for Federal Student Aid (FAFSA)? True, and what a surprise that was for us to learn! According to federal regulations, generally speaking, when a student receives an undergrad degree or reaches the age of 24, he or she is considered independent for FAFSA purposes. But the new reality is that for some nursing grad schools, if you are under the age of 28, you may have to provide parental information. That's why we included a need-to-know financial aid checklist that you can use to help keep you out of harm's way.

We strove to minimize the "gigantic mess," provide the best scholarship resources, reduce loan debt, and guide you through your nursing journey. This comprehensive guide gives nursing students a road map to paying for their advanced nursing degrees. It gives the much-needed direction for navigating the complex problem of paying for advanced nursing degrees. You will learn the secret ins and outs of financing your education from national experts. This guide will enable you to invest in your future profession.

Much success to you in your new career!

Carl Buck
Rick Darvis

ACKNOWLEDGMENTS

First, I would like to thank my business associate Maryann Steffe for her unwavering patience, guidance, and support throughout this project.

In addition, I would like to thank the many friends and colleagues for believing in the value of this book and for their encouragement, including Judy Guy, Kirk Krikstan, Virginia Smith, and Roger Coutant.

Finally, a special thanks to Frank Costanzo and Mary Gatsch at Springer Publishing Company, who reinforced the need for this information for graduate nursing students and embraced this initiative from the onset.

Carl Buck

INTRODUCTION:
A Nurse's Guide on How to Take Ownership of the College Funding Process

This book is meant to be your financial aid advocate. The reality is that a graduate nursing program can be very costly and often results in significant debt. However, it comes with unparalleled personal rewards and career advancements.

Gain insight into three key areas:

- How to overcome unintentional college financial aid barriers and how to manage change

- New financial planning strategies to ensure future financial success

- The latest tax planning innovations for your greatest financial return

Expand your financial aid knowledge base; understand critical deadlines; increase your ability to gain scholarships and grants; and learn how, when, and why to appeal your financial aid award letter.

We will demonstrate innovative revenue concepts and ways to proactively engage the financial aid office. In addition, we will teach you how to own the financial aid process by "partnering" with the graduate financial aid office.

Lastly, if you are studying for your advanced nursing degree and you are also a parent with children who are either going to be in college or already in college, we will show you how that might be a benefit—and not a burden—when it comes to the Free Application for Federal Student Aid (FAFSA) submission.

CHAPTER 1

COLLEGE FUNDING FOR GRADUATE NURSING STUDENTS PROGRAMS

COST AND COMPARISON OF GRADUATE NURSING PROGRAMS

Be selective of costs and comparisons of graduate nursing programs. Research the best programs and schools that fit your needs and budget.

When doing your research for your advanced nursing degree, look for "full transparency." It is critical to shop and compare what your loan debt may be and how long you will need to complete the advanced program.

FULL TRANSPARENCY?
BUYER BEWARE!

What do we mean by *full transparency*? Maybe you remember applying to college as an undergraduate. You looked at the programs offered by colleges, the various activities you could be involved in, and, oh yes, the cost!

Colleges are required to place the full cost of attendance on their website, but I can assure you it is not always easy to find. Next, try to find the average total debt a graduate student will accumulate and how long it will take to obtain that degree; unfortunately, that information is rarely provided—or very difficult to locate.

More than a decade ago, the Higher Education Act of 2008 mandated that colleges provide more transparency on their websites by showing the actual net price that the student would pay. That is when the Net Price Calculator became required to be displayed on each college's website. According to our research for this book, there are many institutions that could use better transparency on their websites that would make the lives of nurses going on for advanced degrees much easier.

In a March 28, 2019, *Inside Higher Ed* article, "Obfuscating Net Price," federal policy reporter Andrew Kreighbaum wrote:

> *Many four-year institutions are failing to meet federal standards for their disclosures more than a decade later, according to a study released . . . by the University of Pennsylvania Graduate School of Education.*[1]

---

1. Kreighbaum, A. (2019). Obfuscating net price. *Inside Higher Ed.* Retrieved from https://insidehighered.com/news/2019/03/28/colleges -fall-short-price-disclosures-study-finds#.XJzW3s7FOAo.email

TOP MSN DEGREE SPECIALTIES

It is interesting to note the following MSN specialties that show both the growth and average salary of these professions. See Table 1.1.

TABLE 1.1 Top MSN Degree Specialties

SPECIALTY	PROJECTED GROWTH BY 2022 (%)	AVERAGE SALARY ($)
Certified Nurse Midwife	31	79,000
Nurse Researcher	26	90,000
Family Nurse Practitioner	25	94,000
Gerontological Nurse Practitioner	25	94,000
Pediatric Nurse Practitioner	25	94,000
Psychiatric Nurse Practitioner	25	94,000
Nurse Anesthetist	22	154,300
Nurse Educator	19	65,000
Pain Management Nurse	19	67,000
Critical Care Nurse	16	61,000

SOURCE: Data from Nurse Journal. (2019). *Top 10 MSN degree specialties.* Retrieved from https://nursejournal.org/msn-degree/top-10-msn-degree-specialities-for-the-future

FUTURE OPPORTUNITIES FOR NURSES WITH ADVANCED DEGREES

Advanced nursing degrees include higher income opportunities, and also offer nurses a variety of positions where they can play a more critical role in patient interaction. With today's population having a longer life expectancy, nurses with advanced degrees will, more likely than not, be able to address concerns such as primary care. It is well known that nurse practitioners have taken on greater roles by assuming the responsibilities that were previously performed by medical doctors.

HAVE YOU CONSIDERED AN ONLINE GRADUATE NURSING PROGRAM?

There is an accelerated growth of online degree programs throughout the country, and graduate nursing degree online programs are no exception. Some online programs allow the graduate nursing student to attend an out-of-state school, but not pay out-of-state tuition, which can minimize debt and provide much more convenience to the student. The good news is that some of the most well-respected colleges are offering online degree programs.

Advantages of online programs include:

- Living costs are significantly lower (no on-campus living required).
- Pacing of program may be adjusted to accelerate or lengthen according to your needs.
- They provide a more comfortable life–work–school balance.

What Nursing Degrees Are Most Commonly Offered Online?

Although some institutions offer a variety of advanced degree online options, some schools may limit their online degrees to a handful of programs. Some of your coursework can be completed online, but the program may also require in-person classroom time. Keep in mind that clinical hours must be taken at a location approved by your school.

How Much Will an Online Advanced Nursing Degree Cost?

According to *U.S. News & World Report* information obtained in 2019, the following schools are ranked as the "Best Online Master's in Nursing Programs":

- Johns Hopkins University: $1,639 per credit
- Ohio State University: $958 per credit for out of state
- St. Xavier University: $750 per credit
- Rush University: $1,066 per credit
- University of Colorado: $655 for out of state
- Duke University: $1,769 per credit
- George Washington University: $1,340 per credit
- Medical University of South Carolina: $1,015 per credit for out of state
- University of South Carolina: $1,403 per credit

- The Catholic University of America: $1,100 per credit
- University of Cincinnati: $655 per credit[2]

NOTE: Scholarships and federal financial aid are available to students enrolled in accredited online degree programs.

TRADITIONAL ON-CAMPUS PROGRAMS

The best on-campus nursing master's programs, as ranked in 2019 according to *U.S. News & World Report,* are:

- Johns Hopkins University
- Duke University
- University of Pennsylvania
- Emory University
- Columbia University
- University of North Carolina–Chapel Hill
- Yale University
- Ohio State University
- Rush University[3]

2. U.S. News & World Report. (2019). Best online master's in nursing programs Retrieved from https://www.usnews.com/education/online -education/nursing/rankings

3. U.S. News & World Report. (2019). *Best nursing schools: Master's.* Retrieved from https://www.usnews.com/best-graduate-schools/top -nursing-schools/nur-rankings

FELLOWSHIP AND RESIDENCY PROGRAMS

Another means of paying for your advanced nursing degree can be found through fellowship and residency programs.

An excerpt from nursejournal.org provides the following information:

> *Nursing students can enhance their educational experience through fellowship and residency programs. These intense, hands-on learning programs provide students with essential nursing skills and also allow students to network with professionals and gain a better understanding of what their responsibilities will be when they begin full-time work. Residency and fellowship programs look great on a graduate's resume and may help students gain future employment. Many programs pair new nurses with mentors who provide professional development support, and both residencies and fellowships may accept undergraduate or graduate students. Most programs offer stipends or salaries to compensate the student. Some residency and fellowship programs may also include an educational award that waives or forgives part of a student's tuition. Residency and fellowship commitments are offered in part-time and full-time formats. These positions may coincide with a student's school attendance or begin shortly after graduation from a nursing program. Fellowships often offer training in a specialty practice area, such as anesthesiology, obstetrics, or psychiatry.*[4]

---

4. Nurse Journal. (n.d.). *Financial aid overview and scholarships: Fellowship and residency programs.* Retrieved from https://nursejournal.org/articles/nursing-scholarships-grants

GRADUATE NURSING STUDENT LOAN DEBT

As you move forward in this book, you will find a variety of options to help minimize your student loan debt. To bring attention to the reality of graduate nursing borrowing, a 2017 report from the American Association of Colleges of Nursing stated:

> *Sixty-nine percent of graduate nursing students surveyed in 2016 took out federal student loans to finance their education. The median amount of student loan debt anticipated by graduate nursing students upon completion of their program was between $40,000 and $54,999. This range captures all graduate levels (i.e., MSN, DNP, PhD) and covers both advanced practice registered nursing (APRN) students (e.g., Certified Registered Nurse Anesthetists, Certified Nurse Midwives, Clinical Nurse Specialists, and Nurse Practitioners) and advanced nursing students. The most significant differences in borrowing habits was that more than half of all students from diverse backgrounds borrowed more than $55,000 to finance their education. This is higher than the total average for the entire sample population.*[5]

---

5. American Association of Colleges of Nursing. (2017). *The numbers behind the degree*. Retrieved from http://www.aacnnursing.org/Portals/42/Policy/PDF/Debt_Report.pdf

CHAPTER 2

THE FINANCIAL AID MAZE

OBTAINING FINANCIAL AID

College financial aid is money coming from a variety of sources such as federal and state governments, schools, local and national organizations, and private lenders, including banks and credit unions.

Free Application for Federal Student Aid

The first step to receiving financial aid is the completion of the infamous Free Application for Federal Student Aid (FAFSA).

If it has been a while since you submitted the FAFSA, you might recall that you had to submit your parent's previous year's tax information if you were a dependent student. And independent students submitted their previous year's tax information as well.

But now . . .

All financial aid applicants must submit their tax information from the prior, prior year. *Got it?*

DIVING INTO THE DETAIL

Applying for undergraduate financial aid was no simple task—and perhaps even more difficult for nurses seeking financial aid for graduate school. Here's why . . .

The financial aid regulations say that when students earn their first undergraduate degree, they are considered independent students for financial aid purposes. This means that when such new "independent" students submit a FAFSA application, they should only be reporting *their*—not the family's—prior, prior year tax information.

However, there could be exceptions. For example, some nursing graduate programs say that if students are under the age of 30, and single, they must report their PARENT'S prior, prior year tax information, even if they are INDEPENDENT students.

That's our opening to alert you on how to navigate a very complex financial aid system. Our experience tells us that no graduate nursing school will necessarily replicate the same financial aid application, nor will funding or financial aid award letters be the same. The FAFSA does have the word *federal* in it, but that can be misleading, as the form can be used for nonfederal aid as well. Some scholarship organizations may request that the FAFSA be submitted to determine which applicant has the most need, in addition to other required scholarship criteria.

The FAFSA could also identify nursing graduate students who might be eligible for institutional need-based loans, apart from federal subsidized or unsubsidized loans.

The new time frame to submit a FAFSA is now October 1, versus the former January 1 timeline. However, it is important to note that nursing graduate students need to check with each nursing program they are applying to for financial aid to determine the priority financial aid filing date for that institution. You can now submit your FAFSA via the myStudentAid mobile app available for iPhone and Android users. It works in conjunction with myFAFSA, which is used to complete the FAFSA.[1]

How Federal Financial Aid Is Determined

The Federal Methodology Formula (FM) is a federal formula used to calculate the expected family contribution (EFC). It is used by every accredited undergraduate, graduate, and trade school in the United States to determine how much federal money can be disbursed by the school to cover the student's Cost of Attendance (COA). Most states also use this formula as a basis to distribute state financial aid funds.

---

1. Financial Aid Toolkit. (2019). *2019–20 FAFSA® Form on myStudent-Aid Mobile App*. Retrieved from https://financialaidtoolkit.ed.gov/tk/announcement-detail.jsp?id=fafsa-mobile-options

Needs Analysis Formula

Needs analysis is the process of determining the financial need of the student. The one thing that hasn't changed in the financial aid world is determining what an applicant is eligible for. Since financial need is the most important factor in determining financial aid, let's see how it is determined. Financial need is calculated using the formula in Box 2.1:

▶ **BOX 2.1   FINANCIAL AID NEEDS ANALYSIS FORMULA**

Cost of attendance (COA) − Expected family contribution (EFC) = Need

For example:

   Cost of Attendance (COA) $25,000

   − Expected Family Contribution (EFC) $7,000

   = Financial Need $18,000

   − Student Resources $1,000

   = Adjusted Financial Need $17,000

   Full COA includes tuition, room and board, books, fees, and so on.

It is interesting to note that some institutions list a loan as a financial aid "award."

WHO GETS NEED-BASED AID?

Need-based grants or scholarships or unsubsidized loans reflect an assessment of the student's ability to pay. They are awarded by the school based on information provided on the FAFSA or any additional supplemental forms required by the institution.

As stated earlier, federal rules do not require students who hold an undergraduate degree to report parental information, regardless of the students' age. However, some graduate nursing programs may require parental FAFSA information up to the age of 30, so be sure to do your research!

As for scholarships, some graduate nursing programs will award both merit and need-based scholarships. Merit scholarships reflect strong academic credentials, and need-based scholarships are based on demonstrated financial need.

FORMS, FORMS, AND MORE FORMS

We have talked about the FAFSA. Now it's time to take an inside look at what additional aid forms might be required by the financial aid office.

As a reminder, your FAFSA will be reporting income, assets, and other related information from two years ago—not the most recent tax year filed. In addition to requiring FAFSA submission, your nursing program may also ask you to complete its own institutional financial aid supplemental form. Once again, make sure to do your research so that your aid application is complete and ready for processing. Many advanced degree nursing programs may require the student to submit separate applications for their scholarship awards, so be sure to check on the scholarships available to you—and the deadline dates.

Nonassessable Assets for Financial Aid Purposes

There are certain nonassessable assets that do not have to be reported on financial aid application forms, and therefore they will not affect the EFC. These items are as follows:

- **Annuities**

  - Annuities (including both qualified and nonqualified annuities) are nonassessable assets.

  - Observation: Some private colleges do assess annuities when computing the EFC. You or your financial adviser should contact each college that you are interested in attending and inquire about its policy regarding assessment of annuities.

- **Life Insurance**

  - Life insurance cash value is not assessed.

  - Observation: Some private colleges do assess life insurance cash value when computing the EFC.

- **Retirement Accounts**

  - Retirement accounts, such as a 401(k), 403(b), IRA, simplified employee pension (SEP), and Keogh, are nonassessable assets. A Roth IRA is also not assessed.

- **Personal Items**

  - Personal items, such as cars, clothes, and household items, are not assessed. Debt corresponding to personal items cannot be listed on the financial aid application forms.

■ **Personal Residence**

▪ The family's primary residence is a nonassessable asset; however, second or vacation homes are assessable assets.

■ **Family Farm or Business**

▪ The family farm or business is a nonassessable asset. A *family farm* is defined as the family's principal place of residence, and the family operates the farm. The *family business* is defined as a business where the family has significant ownership interest and materially participates in its operation. The business must have less than 100 full-time employees. A farm that does not meet the criteria for a family farm is considered an "investment farm" and must be reported at its current market value.

Nonassessable Income

There are certain types of nonassessable income that do not have to be reported on the financial aid application forms and therefore will not affect the EFC. These items are as follows:

■ **Employer-Provided Education Assistance Benefits**

▪ Education assistance benefits received from an employer are not reportable on an employee's financial aid application. However, the amount of the benefit is considered a "resource" and reduces the financial need of the student on a dollar-for-dollar basis.

- **Loan Proceeds**
  - Loan proceeds from any source are not assessed. This would include loans from life insurance, retirement accounts, residences, student loans, and so on.

- **"Rollover" Pensions**
  - The portion of a pension withdrawal, which is not "rolled over" to another type of pension, is assessed; however, any rollover portion is not assessed. For example, if you roll your 401(k) to an IRA, it is a nonassessable rollover.

- **Gifts and Support**
  - Gifts and support, other than money, received from friends or relatives are not assessed. Nonmonetary gifts, such as stocks or automobiles, are not assessed.

- **Veterans Educational Benefits**
  - Veterans Administration (VA) educational benefits, including VA work–study, are not assessed. However, the amount of the benefit is considered a "resource" and reduces the financial need of the student on a dollar-for-dollar basis.

- **Flexible Spending Plan Contributions**
  - Contributions to, or payments from, flexible spending plans are not assessed in the

federal financial aid formula for graduate programs. This includes Medical Savings Accounts (MSAs) and Health Savings Accounts (HSAs). Flexible spending plans increase a student's financial aid eligibility because they reduce the family income.

- *Example:* Families who contributed $8,000 to their flexible spending plans for dependent care and medical expenses reduced their income by the $8,000. This reduction increased the student's financial aid eligibility, because the family income was reduced by this amount.

Assessable Income

There are numerous types of "Untaxed Income and Benefits" that are considered financial aid income.

- **Current Year Retirement Contributions**
  - Deductible IRA, SIMPLE IRA, SEP, or Keogh contributions for the current year are assessed. In addition, payments to tax-deferred pension and savings plans are assessed. This includes the current contributions to 401(k) and 403(b) plans.
  - *Example:* A student—or a parent of a dependent student—made a $3,000 tax-deductible contribution to a regular IRA. The $3,000 is considered an "untaxed benefit" and is used in the EFC computations.
- **Cash received as a gift is considered financial aid income and is assessed.**

- **Untaxed Portion of Retirement Withdrawal**
  - Untaxed portions of retirement, pension, annuity, or life insurance withdrawals, excluding loans, are assessed. This includes distributions from Roth IRAs, whether taxable or nontaxable.
  - The taxable conversion of a regular IRA to a Roth IRA causes an increase in income, so avoid these withdrawals during your graduate studies.

- **Living Allowance**
  - Housing, food, and other living allowances, excluding rent subsidies for low-income housing, paid to members of the military, clergy, and others, including cash payments and cash value benefits, as compensation for their jobs are assessed. For example, if a family receives the tax-free use of an apartment, the rental value of the apartment would be reported. Housing allowances exclude rent subsidies for low-income housing.
  - *Example:* Room and board provided as a nontaxable fringe benefit by a corporation for its employees would be considered an "untaxed benefit."

- **Child Support Payments**
  - Child support payments received for all the children are assessed as untaxed income.
  - Planning tip: A divorce or separation could be structured to give the custodial

parent more assets and smaller child support payments.

■ **Income Exclusions**

▪ Income exclusions, such as the exclusion of the gain on the sale of a personal residence, are assessed. Although these items are not taxable, they must be reported as "untaxed income," as they represent additional financial funds available to the family.

Financial Aid Deductions

Taxable Grants and Scholarships

Taxable grant and scholarship aid that is included in the student's taxable income is a deduction against the student's income for federal tax purposes.

Federal Income Tax

Federal income tax paid—actual tax paid, not the amount withheld—is a deduction on financial aid income. This does not include Social Security tax on tips, the 10% penalty on early withdrawals from retirement accounts, the advance earned income credit, or household employment taxes.

State Tax Allowance

An allowance for state tax is a deduction. This is automatically calculated by the financial aid processing center in the financial aid formula, based on the state of residency.

Social Security Tax

Social Security tax paid is a deduction. This is automatically calculated by the financial aid processing center based on the amount of earned income of the parents and student.

Keeping Yourself Organized

Develop a spreadsheet that covers the financial aid deadline dates and other requirements (Table 2.1).

TABLE 2.1 Example of Financial Aid Spreadsheet

	SCHOOL NAME	SCHOOL NAME	SCHOOL NAME
Application Due Date			
Misc. Documents Required			
Scholarship Application Due Date			
Full Cost of Attendance—campus			
Full Cost of Attendance—online			
Merit Scholarships Offered			
Need-Based Grants Offered			

(continued)

TABLE 2.1 (*Continued*)

	SCHOOL NAME	SCHOOL NAME	SCHOOL NAME
GPA Required to Maintain Scholarships & Grants			
Total Time for Advanced Degree Completion			
Total Projected Debt at Graduation			
NOTES			

Understanding Your Financial Aid Award: Did You Get a Good Deal?

Let's review the actual financial aid award given to a student, Julia, 24 years old, accepted to a private School of Nursing to pursue her MSN. Julia is an independent student for financial aid purposes, due to the fact that she has her BSN and is 24 years old (Tables 2.2–2.5).

TABLE 2.2 Cost of Attendance

Budget Category	Amount	COA
Tuition	$84,700	Your COA is based on attendance for the first 12 months of your program. The amounts shown are to help you plan for the academic year. This includes direct costs such as tuition, university fees, and health insurance and indirect costs such as books and supplies, transportation, and personal expenses. Students with their own health insurance may waive the student health insurance. These figures are a conservative and modest estimate of living expenses for all students. Students do not need to borrow for expenses outlined, but may do so under federal regulations.
Network Fee	$585	
Program Fee	$150	
Simulation Lab Fee	$75	
Student Activity Fee	$105	
Technology Fee	$150	
Transcript Fee	$105	
Health Insurance Fee	$3,968	
Student Health Fees	$1,787	
Room & Board	$27,840	
Books & Supplies	$2,050	
Transportation	$1,452	**Anticipated Cost of Attendance for Final Term**
Personal Expenses	$2,808	As the final summer term is part of the 2020–2021 academic year, we are providing you with an estimated cost of attendance for the final 3 months of the program. The estimated cost of tuition and fees is $28,865 (this does not include indirect cost).
Loan Fee	$2,570	

Budget Totals	$128,345	

COA, cost of attendance.

TABLE 2.3 School of Nursing Grants Awarded

	TOTAL	SCHOOL OF NURSING MERIT SCHOLARSHIP:
Institution Grant(s)		To be eligible for the Merit Scholarship, students must be
Merit Scholarship	$15,000	enrolled full-time (or following your program plan) and in good
Need Scholarship	$28,510	academic standing. Students on academic or behavioral probation
	--------	risk forfeiting any grant funding.
Total Grant(s)	$43,510	Students who take a Leave of Absence, which is not required by program, forfeit their scholarship on return. This award will be reevaluated each academic term.
		SCHOOL OF NURSING NEED SCHOLARSHIP: The Need Scholarship is a need-based scholarship. This scholarship will be adjusted if a student no longer has an educational financial need. Students who receive funding to cover their needs must provide documentation of the new funding to the Office of Financial Aid to still be eligible to receive the scholarship. All students must report personal financial changes that may affect their scholarship or loan eligibility to the Office of Financial Aid. To be eligible for the Need Scholarship, students must be enrolled full-time (or following your program plan) and in good academic standing. Students on academic or behavioral probation risk forfeiting any grant funding. Students who take a Leave of Absence, which is not required during the program, forfeit their scholarship on return. This award will be reevaluated each academic term.

TABLE 2.4 Loans Awarded

LOANS	TOTAL	FEDERAL DIRECT UNSUBSIDIZED LOAN: Students offered a Federal Direct Unsubsidized Loan may borrow up to the amount indicated on this award letter over the course of the academic year.
Federal Direct Unsubsidized Loan	$20,500	
Total	$20,500	This loan is borrowed through the U.S. Department of Education, is not based on financial needs, and you are responsible for all interest accrued while you are enrolled in school and during approved periods of grace and deferment.
		For the 2019–20 school year, the interest rate is fixed at 6.08% for Graduate Students. Loan repayment begins 6 months after you graduate or cease to be enrolled at least half time. Loans disbursed after October 1, 2018 will carry an origination fee of 1.062%, as of this writing.

TABLE 2.5 2019–20 Awards Breakdown by Term

AWARDS Source	Summer 2019	Fall 2019	Spring 2020	Total
Merit Scholarship	$0	$7,500	$7,500	$15,000
Need Scholarship	$0	$14,255	$14,255	$28,510
Federal Direct Unsubsidized Loan	$6,834	$6,833	$6,833	$20,500
Alternative Eligibility (Loans)	$33,360	$13,767	$17,208	$64,335
Total	$40,194	$42,355	$45,796	$128,345

ALTERNATIVE ELIGIBILITY

Alternative eligibility is the difference between your cost of attendance and the aid awarded. This may be met with loans from credit-based educational loan programs (Federal Direct Graduate PLUS and private), personal or family resources, or savings. For loans that are credit-based, it is important to apply as soon as possible to ensure that funding will be available.

PLANNING CONSIDERATIONS

It appears that this private institution expects this student to borrow about $85,000, based on the award letter, but this is based on 8 months of a 12-month program. This student needs to determine the additional FULL cost of attendance for the remaining 3 months, and how much more debt will be incurred.

What the student needs to know from the financial aid office:

1. What was the EFC from the FAFSA?

2. Based on the fact that the student will have to take out two loans to pay the bill, the student should appeal to the financial aid office for additional grant, and/or merit scholarship, funding for the student to enroll.

3. Get information about nursing loan forgiveness programs.

4. As the final summer term is part of the 2020–21 academic year, the university provided an estimated cost of attendance for

the final 3 months of the program. The estimated cost of tuition and fees is $28,865 (this does not include indirect costs).

5. The graduate student should request the anticipated FULL cost of attendance for the remaining 3 months of the MSN program and ask if the university would provide any aid—need based or nonneed based—assistance for that term.

Appealing a Financial Aid Award

When a college's award letter does not meet the student's financial needs, either in the total amount of aid or in the type of aid, the student can appeal the award to the college. Most colleges have an appeal process that allows students to request a review of their financial aid eligibility and a corresponding financial aid award offer. Each college determines its own regulations for this process, and students should be aware of a particular college's procedures.

▶ **PLANNING TIP 1**

If the student does appeal an award letter, the student should be specific in requesting additional funds. The student should clearly state the reasons for the appeal and request a specific amount of money. The student should write the request and submit any required documents with a letter of appeal. Then, the student should contact the college's financial aid administrator (FAA). It is preferable to make contact in person; if this is not possible, the administrator should be contacted by a telephone call. The "personal touch" is important to a successful appeal.

Professional Judgment

In the appeal letter, the student should ask the FAA to exercise "professional judgment." Professional judgment is the authority given to the college FAA to change the family's financial and household data in any way that would more accurately measure the family's ability to pay for educational costs. If the student is to successfully appeal an award letter, he or she must fully understand the concept and definition of professional judgment. Professional judgment may be exercised only in special circumstances, and only when the family provides adequate documentation of these special circumstances.

Special Circumstances

Special circumstances that are considered for financial aid purposes include unusual medical or dental expenses, dislocated worker, unemployed worker, or unusually high childcare expenses. It could also include circumstances that were considered to be "special conditions," such as divorce, separation, or the death of spouse; or natural disasters (e.g., floods, fires, hurricane, earthquake), after the application was filed. If these situations occur, the college's FAA should be contacted to see whether the aid award can be increased.

Professional judgment can also be used by the FAA in other situations as follows:

1. Adjust the college cost of attendance to take into account special circumstances

such as medical needs or excessive travel costs.

2. Override the student's dependency status to make a "dependent student" an "independent student."

3. Adjust the income and assets of a family located in a federally declared natural disaster area.

    Example: A family, residing in a county that was declared a Federal Natural Disaster Area due to flooding, appealed the income and asset amounts reported on the FAFSA to the FAA at the college the student was attending. The family documented that the value of the building, which contained the family business, had been greatly reduced due to damages sustained during the flood. The family did not have flood insurance to cover the damage. Also, the family's income generated by the business assets would be greatly reduced during the upcoming period of clean-up and repair. The FAA agreed that this was indeed a special circumstance and adjusted the student's original FAFSA amounts and increased the amount of the original financial aid award.

4. Any other "special circumstance" that the family and/or its financial adviser can supply to convince the FAA to adjust the EFC data elements.

    Example: A student was able to convince the FAA that his "un-reimbursed business expenses" would reduce his income because they were actually "out-of-pocket" expenses against his income.

Example: A student demonstrated to the FAA that her employment projected year income would be much less during graduate school than was reported on the FAFSA.

Award Letter Strategies

1. Check the deadline date for acceptance of the award letter.

2. Check the EFC on the award letter (if it is shown) with the EFC shown on the Student Aid Report (SAR) to check the accuracy of EFC shown on the award letter.

3. Make sure the "true COA" is indicated on the award letter. If a COA is not shown or it appears to leave out some costs, determine the "true COA."

4. Federal Grad PLUS Loans or Federal Direct Unsubsidized Loans should be considered as financial aid possibilities; they both have very favorable interest rates and the interest could be tax deductible.

5. Determine whether the grant and scholarship aid are renewable and the criteria for renewal.

6. Accepting an award letter does not prevent the student from filing a future appeal of the award letter.

7. When all the award letters have been received, the student should compare them to determine the best award; that is, less loan

debt versus free money and duration of the program.

8. If the award letter does not meet the expectations of the student, it should be appealed to the FAA. Find out whether the appeal can be based on any special circumstances unique to the student's situation.

CHAPTER 3

PAYING FOR YOUR ADVANCED NURSING DEGREE

LOANS FOR COLLEGE

Education loans for advanced nursing degrees come in the following categories:

- Federal Direct Unsubsidized Student Loan
- Federal Direct Grad PLUS Loan
- Nursing student loan
- Private education loan

FEDERAL DIRECT LOANS

Federal Direct Student Loans are a form of financial aid that must be repaid with interest. The school determines the amount you can borrow based on your cost of attendance (COA) and other aid you receive.

Subsidized loans are based on financial need; unsubsidized loans are nonneed based. However, both types of loans have an origination fee deducted from the loan amount at the time of disbursement. These loans have low fixed interest rates for the life of the loan; interest rates are set by federal law and historically change on July 1 (either higher or lower) for new loans. A graduate or professional student can borrow up to $20,500 in Direct Unsubsidized Loans and up to $138,500 aggregate amount. "Graduate and professional students enrolled in certain health profession programs may receive additional Direct Unsubsidized Loan amounts each academic year . . . For these students, there is also a higher aggregate limit on Direct Unsubsidized Loans. If you are enrolled in a health profession program, talk to the financial aid office at your school for information about annual and aggregate limits."[1]

Benefits of the Federal Direct Loan:

- Fixed interest rate for the life of the loan
- If financial need is determined, the student may qualify for subsidized loans, and the government pays the interest while the student is enrolled at least half-time.
- Deferment option on unsubsidized loans
- Six-month grace period before repayment begins when the student graduates, leaves school, or drops below half-time enrollment

---

1. Federal Student Aid. (n.d.). Types of aid: Loans: Subsidized and unsubsidized loans. Retrieved from https://studentaid.ed.gov/sa/types/loans/subsidized-unsubsidized

- Flexible repayment plans (check with the financial aid office for further information)
- Loan forgiveness for qualified circumstances (check with the financial aid office)[2]

GRAD PLUS LOAN

Grad PLUS is a federal loan also funded by the Department of Education (ED) and has benefits similar to those of Federal Direct Loans. Eligibility for the Grad PLUS Loan is determined by completing the FAFSA but is not based on financial need; however, a credit check is required. Assuming that you do not have adverse credit history, as a graduate or professional student you can borrow up to the cost of education minus any other financial aid (e.g., scholarships, grants). If you cannot document the extenuating circumstances or fix your credit issues, you may need to have a cosigner on the loan. An origination fee is charged on this loan.

NURSING STUDENT LOANS

Students should check with the financial aid office to determine if the institution offers its own nursing student loan program.

"The Health Resources and Services Administration (HRSA) provides funding to participating schools to offer long-term, low-interest loans to full-time, disadvantaged students pursuing a diploma, associate, baccalaureate or

2. Federal Direct Loan. (2019). Retrieved from https://studentaid .ed.gov/sa/types/loans

graduate degree in nursing."[3] Find out if your school participates in the Nursing Student Loan program at https://bhw.hrsa.gov/loans-scholarships/school-based-loans.

PRIVATE EDUCATION LOANS

Private education loans are nonfederal loans, made by a private lender such as a bank, credit union, or state agency, and there are no federal forms to complete. In some cases, private loan interest rates may be as competitive as those for a Federal Direct Grad PLUS Loan.

The advantage to a nurse choosing a private loan is the competitive interest rates. There are usually no loan application fees or origination fee. Variable and fixed rates may be lower than the Federal Direct Grad PLUS Loans.

However, federal education loans may offer better repayment and forgiveness options. Thus, students should consider exhausting their eligibility for federal education loans before considering private student loans.

Private loans do not offer income-based repayment options and may not offer deferment or forbearance options.

PERSONAL RESIDENCE AND HOME EQUITY LOANS

Graduate students who consider using private education loans often also consider using a personal residence

---

3. Health Resources and Services Administration. (n.d.). School-based loans and scholarships. Retrieved from https://bhw.hrsa.gov/loans-scholarships/school-based-loans

or home equity loan to finance their education. *Home equity* is the difference between the fair market value of your home and what you owe on it. In other words, it is the portion of the total value of your house that you already own. Although many families do not want to mortgage their home to pay for college costs, it may be a better source of funds than borrowing on their business assets or from their retirement accounts. Another consideration is the fees you may pay for a loan. Fees are simply another loan cost in addition to interest, and as such, all education loans being considered should be compared by calculating the equivalent interest rate and fees (if there are any) of each loan. If the student (or family) uses a home equity line of credit (LOC) to fund college, he or she can borrow what is needed as and when it is needed. Therefore, the student will pay interest on only the amount borrowed. Persons with loans are usually allowed to make minimum monthly payments and can then make larger payments after they are done with college. Another strategic advantage of paying for college with a home equity loan is the fact that proceeds from a home equity LOC used for education are not considered "income" in the financial aid formula. However, if the student (or family) refinances, or uses a second mortgage to fund college, he or she will borrow a fixed, lump sum amount that probably will not be used all at once, and the student will be paying interest on money not currently needed. Therefore, the student should consider investing the excess funds in a short-term investment until the funds are needed for college. (For parents/students whose income is too high [modified adjusted gross income (MAGI) is less than $75,000 ($155,000 if filing a joint return)] to take advantage of the student loan interest deduction, a personal residence loan can give them an itemized income tax deduction [subject to the rules for high income]. This deduction is not limited to $2,500, as is the case for student loan interest.)

The repayment term on residence loans is usually longer than retirement account loans and other types of loans, which makes the monthly payments smaller.

▶ **PLANNING TIP 1**

For conservative long-term investors, aggressively prepaying their home mortgage to avoid high interest costs can pay big dividends as a college and retirement strategy. The longer the client stays in a home, the larger the cash flow savings. Working with a certified financial adviser is highly recommended.

RETIREMENT ACCOUNT LOANS

Borrowing from retirement accounts may be considered as a source for college funding. The advantages of borrowing from these sources are a generally favorable interest rate and repayment terms and ease of obtaining the loan. However, if these loans are not repaid within a certain period of time, usually 5 years, the outstanding principal balance becomes taxable income and subject to a 10% penalty if the borrower is under age 59½.

Also, if the employee loses a job, the outstanding loan balance may have to be immediately repaid, or taxable income occurs. In addition, the borrower gives up the ability to defer tax on the withdrawn assets and may be jeopardizing retirement savings.

Furthermore, even though the retirement fund earns interest on the college loan, it foregoes the interest it would have earned had it been invested in a mutual fund at a possibly higher rate of return.

Some retirement plans prohibit or restrict distributions before retirement. However, hardship distributions from 401(k) plans (subject to the 10% penalty) are allowed to meet certain college expenses. Taking a hardship distribution precludes the plan participant from contributing to the plan for 12 months.

LIFE INSURANCE LOANS

Life insurance loans can be another source of graduate school funding. The student should beware of taking out a life insurance loan. What typically happens when one takes out a life insurance loan for a long period of time is that the loan balance increases, because the borrower doesn't pay the interest. Therefore, as the loan value increases, the death benefits become less, if any. Also, the loan balance can eat up all the cash value, and there is no cash left in the policy to sustain it. The policy then terminates unless the client pays back the loan. If it terminates, the client doesn't have to repay the loan plus accrued interest but then has to recognize this as taxable income.

If the student is borrowing from the policy for college expense and doesn't plan on repayment, the client should only borrow an amount that will not terminate the policy until age 100, taking into account whether interest and premiums will be paid out of pocket or not. The loan is usually paid off on death out of the proceeds. Life insurance loans can give the client an option of paying for college, but the student should beware of the pitfalls of borrowing too much and causing the policy to terminate.

INTRAFAMILY LOANS

Generally, a disparity exists between the rate of earnings on an investment and the interest rate a borrower must pay on a loan. Loaning money to a student for college costs can offer savings opportunities for both the parent and the student. The parents may be able to both increase their rate of return on investments and assist their child in paying for college. The child may increase cash flow for college, due to the lower interest rate on the loan than could be obtained from other financing.

Note: The interest paid on loans from relatives is not deductible as student loan interest expense.

Example: The parents have $150,000 in their savings account that earns 5% annually. Their child needs $125,000 for college; however, the 9% rate the child needs to pay to a lending institution is higher than the child would like. The parents want to loan the student the money, but they need the income generated from their savings account to live on. The parties agree on a 7% interest rate on the loan. The parent's marginal tax rate is 25% and the child's tax rate is 10% to 15%. In this case, the parents will have an increased earnings of $2,500 ([7% − 5%] × $125,000), less the increased tax liability of $625, or a net after-tax increase of cash flow to $1,875. The student will have a decreased interest expense of $2,500 ([9% − 7%] × [$125,000]. The combined increase in family cash flow is $4,375 ($1,875 + $2,500).

PENSION PLAN

Try borrowing from your 401(k) plan or a pension plan. Many plans will allow you to borrow up to 50% of the value of the plan or up to $50,000 interest-free.

NURSING LOAN FORGIVENESS PROGRAMS

The U.S. ED sponsors a general loan forgiveness program that nurses qualify for. To receive loan forgiveness, the borrower must make 120 monthly payments and hold a full-time public service job, or work for a nonprofit, during that 10-year period. Public health positions such as nurses, nurse practitioners, and nurses in a clinical setting fulfill the public service job requirement. Check the program's specifications to ensure that your loans qualify: https://studentaid.ed.gov/sa/repay-loans/forgiveness-cancellation/public-service#qualify.

As stated in the following excerpt from an article written by Jennifer Wadia for the Student Debt Relief website, "*Thanks to state-specific and federal initiatives, nurses have access to some of the best student loan forgiveness programs out there. Some offer forgivable loans to help offset your initial college costs while others offer loan forgiveness following graduation. If you are a nurse, find out what programs you qualify for based on where you live and the type of loans you have.*[4] *See the link in the footnote to learn about 50 different programs for student loan forgiveness for nurses.*

LOAN CONSOLIDATION

A consolidation loan is designed to help student and parent borrowers simplify loan repayment by allowing the borrower to consolidate several types of federal student loans with various repayment schedules into one loan.[5] Even one loan can be consolidated into a Direct Consolidation Loan to get benefits such as flexible repayment options. If the borrower has more than one loan, a consolidation loan simplifies the repayment process because there is only one payment per month. Also, the interest rate on the consolidation loan may be lower than what is currently being paid on one or more loans.

There is no application fee to consolidate your federal education loans into a Direct Consolidation Loan. If you are contacted by someone offering to consolidate your loans for a fee, you are not dealing with one of the U.S. ED's consolidation servicers.

---

4. Wadia, J. (2019). Student loan forgiveness for nurses. *Student Debt Relief.* Retrieved from https://www.studentdebtrelief.us/student-loan -forgiveness/for-nurses

5. Federal Student Aid. (n.d.). How to repay your loans: Loan consolidation. Retrieved from https://studentaid.ed.gov/sa/repay-loans/con solidation#interest-rate

Should I Consolidate My Loans?

Carefully consider whether loan consolidation is the best option for you. Loan consolidation can greatly simplify loan repayment by centralizing your loans to one bill and can lower monthly payments by giving you up to 30 years to repay your loans. You might also have access to alternative repayment plans you would not have had before. And you will be able to switch your variable interest rate loans to a fixed interest rate.

However, if you increase the length of your repayment period, you will also make more payments and pay more in interest. Be sure to compare your current monthly payments with what monthly payments would be if you consolidated your loans.

If you want to lower your monthly payment amount but are concerned about the impact of loan consolidation, you can consider deferment or forbearance as options for short-term payment relief needs. Once your loans are combined into a Direct Consolidation Loan, they cannot be separated or reinstated. The loans that were consolidated are paid off and no longer exist.

What Types of Loans Can Be Consolidated?

The following education loans are eligible for consolidation:

- Direct Subsidized Loans
- Direct Unsubsidized Loans

- Direct PLUS Loans
- Federal Perkins
- Federal Nursing Loans
- Health Education Assistance Loans
- Some existing consolidation loans

Note: Private education loans are not eligible for a Direct Consolidation Loan.

What Are the Requirements to Consolidate a Loan?

You must have at least one Federal Direct Loan that is in a grace period, or in repayment. If you want to consolidate a defaulted loan, you must either make satisfactory repayment arrangements on the loan with your current loan servicer before you consolidate, or you must agree to repay your new Direct Consolidation Loan under one of the following three plans:

1. Income-based repayment plan
2. Pay as you earn repayment plan
3. Income-contingent repayment plan

Generally, you cannot consolidate an existing consolidation loan again, unless you include an additional Federal Direct Loan, or Federal Family Education Loan (FFEL) Program loan, in the consolidation.

There are no application fees for a Direct Consolidation Loan, and you may prepay your loan at any time without penalty.

What Is the Interest Rate on a Federal Direct Consolidation Loan?

A Direct Consolidation Loan has a fixed interest rate for the life of the loan. The fixed rate is based on the weighted average of the interest rates on the loans being consolidated, rounded up to the nearest one-eighth of 1%. There is no cap on the interest rate of a Direct Consolidation Loan.[6]

When Do I Begin Repayment?

Repayment of a Direct Consolidation Loan can begin 60 days after the loan is disbursed, or sooner. Your loan servicer will let you know when the first payment is due. The repayment term ranges from 10 to 30 years, depending on the amount of your consolidation loan, your other education loan debt, and the repayment plan you select. Note: If any loan you want to consolidate is still in the grace period, you can delay entering repayment on your new Direct Consolidation Loan until closer to your grace period end date. You will indicate this when you apply, and the consolidation servicer will wait to process your application until the appropriate time.

---

6. Federal Student Aid. (n.d.). How to repay your loans: Loan consolidation: What is the interest rate on a consolidation loan? Retrieved from https://studentaid.ed.gov/sa/repay-loans/consolidation#interest-rate

How Do I Apply for a Direct Consolidation Loan?

You apply for a Direct Consolidation Loan through StudentLoans.gov. Once you sign in to StudentLoans.gov using your personal identifiers and Federal Student Aid PIN, you will be able to electronically complete the Federal Direct Consolidation Loan Application and Promissory Note.

After you submit your application electronically via StudentLoans.gov or by mailing a paper application, the consolidation servicer selected will complete the actions required to consolidate your eligible loans. The consolidation servicer will be your point of contact for any questions you may have related to your consolidation application.

It is critical that you continue repayment, if required, to the holders or servicers of the loans you want to consolidate until your consolidation servicer informs you that the underlying loans have been paid off.

▶ **PLANNING TIP 2**

Federal rules stipulate that the student can only consolidate student loans once. There is one way around the rule, but it means taking on even more debt. The government allows students to refinance consolidated student loans, but only if the student has a new student loan—or one that was never consolidated in the first place—to include in the consolidation. If, for example, a student consolidated his or her loans 5 years ago, and then took out a new loan this year to pay for career-related courses, the student may be eligible to consolidate both loans.

> ▶ **PLANNING TIP 3**
>
> If the student plans to borrow for graduate school, he or she can consolidate the undergraduate loans during his or her grace period, and defer payment on the combined loan upon returning to graduate school. That will leave the student the option of consolidating any graduate school loans down the road.

> ▶ **PLANNING TIP 4**
>
> If the student is extremely strapped for cash, he or she could extend the repayment period as well as reduce the interest rate. This may reduce the monthly tab by as much as half.

STUDENT LOAN REPAYMENT

It's not unusual for nursing students going on for advanced degrees to have to take out more than one loan at the same time and with different interest rates. In addition, there may be an undergraduate loan that also might be deferred due to a nurse going on for his or her master's or doctorate.

Let's take an up-close and personal look at a **real case:** Nursing master's degree candidate Beverly (not her real name) is excited to learn she has been admitted to a top nursing school program in the East. Not only did she get admitted, but she also was offered $40,000 in free grant money: $25,000 in need-based grant money and $15,000 in merit scholarship funds. A pretty good deal so far.

Time to dig into the award letter and determine how much the total master's program costs and how far the $40,000 free grant funds will go to pay the full cost of attendance.

The master's nursing program at this East Coast school will cost approximately $128,000 for a year-and-a-half program. When you do the math, cost of attendance is $128,000 minus $43,000 (grants) = a balance due of $85,000.

Yes, $85,000 due, which means that this nursing student will need to borrow $85,000 in loans from a Federal Direct Unsubsidized Loan and a Grad PLUS Loan. As stated earlier, this grad student will have to get two loans, with loan fees to factor in as well. An enormous debt to repay!

What alternatives can be considered? First, Beverly should appeal to the financial aid office to see if the $15,000 merit award can be increased based on her undergrad grades. The need component of her award ($28,000) cannot be appealed due to her $0 expected family contribution.

Alternative Loan Repayment Options
Income Share Agreement

- Borrowing to pay for an advanced nursing degree is to be expected, in almost all cases. But what if you didn't have to borrow and instead "agreed" to accept tuition funds from an investor such as a college or an independent company?

■ *Income Shared Agreements (ISAs) work like this:*

  ▪ A nursing student agrees to accept a certain amount of ISA funds and in return pays back the agreed amount based on future employment earnings. Like all business transactions/agreements, ISAs must be researched and (most importantly) compared and understood, but an ISA might be the right financial fit.

Credit Union Refinancing

■ We don't want to leave out credit union options when considering either borrowing for college or refinancing your student loans.

■ Our experience has shown that a loan from a credit union may offer you a lower interest rate than a loan from a private lender.

■ If you are looking to refinance your student loans—loans from various lenders, including the federal government—credit unions could be a strong choice; however, you can lose some federal loan benefits such as loan forgiveness and grace periods. Once again, understand what you are agreeing to, both positive and negative. No one said this is easy.

■ Finally, you may want to check out credit union student choice. Credit union student choice is more like an umbrella credit union, meaning they are associated with multiple credit unions and offer free college financial aid phone counseling by appointment.

POSTPONING EDUCATION LOANS: LOAN DEFERMENT

A *deferment* is a period during which repayment of the principal and interest of your loan is temporarily delayed.

WHO QUALIFIES FOR A LOAN DEFERMENT?

The student qualifies for deferment of the student loans when the student meets one of the following six criteria:

1. The student must be enrolled, at least half time, at an institution that meets the eligibility requirements for a particular loan.

2. The student must be enrolled in a graduate fellowship program, or a rehabilitation training program for the disabled.

3. The student must be unemployed (for up to 3 years), but actively seeking employment.

4. The student is facing economic hardship (for up to 3 years). Economic hardship includes a broad range of reasons that enable the student to defer the loans.

5. The student is in a period of active duty military service during a war, military operation, or national emergency.

6. The student is in the 13-month period following the conclusion of qualifying active duty

military service, or until the student returns to enrollment on at least a half-time basis, whichever is earlier.

WHAT HAPPENS TO MY LOAN DURING DEFERMENT?

During a deferment, you do not need to make payments. What is more, depending on the type of loan you have, the federal government may pay the interest on your loan during a period of deferment.

The government pays the interest on your Federal Perkins Loans and Federal Direct Subsidized Loans.

The government does not pay the interest on your unsubsidized loans and PLUS loans. You are responsible for paying the interest that accrues (accumulates) during the deferment period, but your payment is not due during the deferment period. If you do not pay the interest on your loan during deferment, it may be capitalized (added to your principal balance), and the amount you pay in the future will be higher.

HOW DO I REQUEST A DEFERMENT?

The procedure for obtaining a loan deferment is simple, but many deferments are not automatic. You will likely need to submit a request to your loan servicer, the organization that handles your loan account. If you are enrolled in school, at least half-time, and you would like to request an in-school deferment, you will need to contact your school's financial aid office, as well as your loan servicer.

Your deferment request should be submitted to the organization to which you make your loan payments.

- Federal Direct Loans and FFEL program loans: contact your loan servicer.

- Perkins loans: contact the school you were attending when you received the loan.

INTRODUCTION TO PAYING OFF LOANS

During college years many people hunker down and tighten their belts. They cut back on their spending and may have less income coming in.

Are you looking for ways to cut costs during these difficult economic times?

Are you looking for ways to reduce the time it takes to pay off your student debt?

If so, there's one surefire way that you can cut costs, and at the same time get a guaranteed rate of return on your money: pay off your outstanding debt and the ridiculously high finance charges that go along with that debt.

Are you aware of how much your debt really costs you? Let's take a closer look:

Example: The Smiths recently refinanced their home to take out money to purchase a new car. Their new mortgage was $316,500 at a fixed rate of 6.5% for 30 years. Exhibit 3.1 is a sample of their Truth-In-Lending Disclosure Statement that comes with every mortgage.

EXHIBIT 3.1   SAMPLE OF A TRUTH-IN-LENDING DISCLOSURE STATEMENT

Loan Number: 0052789478

FEDERAL TRUTH-IN-LENDING DISCLOSURE STATEMENT

(Real Estate)

Lender (Creditor)　　　　　　　　　Borrower(s) Name(s)

Option One Mortgage Co.　　　　　　John Doe

2600 Corporate Exchange Drive　　　Salle Doe

City, State, 45000

　　　　　　　　　　　　　　　　　Address

Loan Type: Conventional　　　　　　10105 State Street

　　　　　　　　　　　　　　　　　City, State, 52000

ANNUAL PERCENTAGE RATE	FINANCE CHARGE	AMOUNT FINANCED	TOTAL OF PAYMENTS
The cost of your credit as a yearly rate	The dollar amount the credit will cost you	The amount of credit provided to your or on your behalf	The amount you will have paid after you made all payments as scheduled
6.500%	**$403,678**	**$316,500**	**$720,178**

Over the next 30 years the Smiths will pay $403,678 in total finance charges for that mortgage, effectively paying for their home more than twice ($720,178/$316,500)!

If the Smiths could afford to make extra payments on their mortgage, they could dramatically reduce the amount they end up paying for their home. Yet, most people feel that they can't afford to make extra payments toward their debt. They need all the money they can get.

However, that's not true! You can have your cake and eat it too. You can pay off your debt faster and you can do it with minimal changes in your current spending habits or financial lifestyle!

How?

You can use the following loan repayment system to pay off your debt in a fraction of the time, while dramatically reducing your interest expense and increasing your credit rating (FICO score) at the same time.

You can virtually become completely debt free in record time with little or no financial impact on your day-to-day spending habits.

Most families use their checking account to deposit their income and pay their monthly expenses. At the end of the month, any money that the family has left over is either left in their checking account or transferred into a savings account.

Most Americans carry a monthly checking account balance from $1,000 to $10,000. Some families carry balances of as much as $50,000 to $100,000, and even more. However, this excess money sits in those checking and savings accounts earning very little money. Most have a rate of return of ... 0%!

This traditional method of handling money can be very expensive if the family builds up significant balances in their checking and savings accounts, while carrying substantial balances on their mortgage and credit cards with finance charges ranging from 6% to 20%, and even more!

Think of it this way: Why would you keep money in a checking or savings account that earns you a rate of return of 0%, when you can use that money to get a guaranteed rate of return of 6% to 20% or more by paying off your mortgage or credit cards and avoiding the high finance charges?

The answer is simple. The reason most families keep large balances in their personal checking accounts is to create a financial reserve in case of emergencies. However, this loan repayment concept allows you to do both:

- Keep a financial reserve in case of emergencies, and
- Use the excess money in your checking or savings account to reduce debt

How can this be done?

It's done by the creative use of a bank LOC.

All loans work on the declining balance method. This means that as payments are made, the finance charges (interest) are taken out, and the balance of the payment is applied against the remaining principal of the loan. It's the gradual reduction of this principal that reduces your debt to zero.

Conventional mortgages, business loans, and student loans are all "closed-end" loan vehicles, meaning there is a set period of time during which you make standard payments. This is called an *amortization schedule*. Once payments are made over that time period, the loan is then paid off.

An "open-end" LOC is similar to a revolving LOC (credit card). A borrower goes to a bank (lender) and establishes an LOC. This LOC can be a secured LOC (home equity LOC), or an unsecured LOC.

The LOC also has a feature that other loan vehicles do not have: the borrower has the flexibility to use any amount of the LOC when he or she needs it, and only pay finance charges on the amount she or he uses. In other words, the borrower can take out a $25,000 LOC, keep $13,000 as a "reserve" that can be used anytime for emergencies, and only pay finance charges on the $12,000 that was actually used.

Furthermore, some banks allow you to deposit money (such as your paycheck) into and write checks (to pay your bills) out of these open-end loan vehicles. In essence, this LOC account becomes your checking account.

Therefore, depending on the timing of these deposits and check payments, and the excess money you carry in the LOC account, the average daily balance (and the interest you pay on that balance) can be greatly reduced over time. As the monthly interest payment due on an LOC is based on the outstanding balance, no monthly finance charges due if the LOC has a zero balance.

The fundamental strategy involving the loan repayment process is to get you to use your idle cash to work more efficiently for you. To do this you simply shift the balance of your excess cash from a low-return bank account to reduce the interest expense (finance charges) of your higher-cost mortgage or other debt account.

Exhibit 3.2 explains how the simple cash flow maximizer process works.

EXHIBIT 3.2 HOW THE CASH FLOW MAXIMIZER STRATEGY WORKS

1. The excess money you carry in your checking or savings account does not work very efficiently when it earns little or no interest or rate of return.

2. If you used that idle, or excess, money to pay down your mortgage or credit cards, it would be the same as getting a 6%–20% rate of return on that money.

3. Most people feel comfortable carrying a cash reserve for emergencies, even if it earns 0%.

4. If you could use your mortgage as your checking account that you could deposit money into and write checks from, any excess money would gradually reduce your debt and the finance charges you pay on your mortgage.

5. You can't do this with your closed-end mortgage, so you use an "open-end" LOC account that functions as your primary checking account. Then you begin the process by advancing a predetermined lump sum from the LOC account and applying it to your mortgage account.

(continued)

EXHIBIT 3.2 (*Continued*)

6. At the same time you continue to make your normal monthly mortgage payments.

7. Together, these payments dramatically reduce the mortgage balance you owe and thus, the finance charges you pay.

8. Then, you continue to use the LOC account as your checking account to deposit money and write checks, while also providing you with an available cash reserve for emergencies.

9. Any excess money (deposits minus checks) that you carry in the LOC account will gradually reduce the LOC balance you owe to $0.

10. Then, you repeat this entire process over and over until your debt is paid free and clear.

Example: Each month John receives a $7,000 paycheck and writes $6,000 in checks to cover his bills, including his mortgage. His monthly excess cash flow is $1,000. John takes out an LOC of $25,000, keeps $13,000 in his LOC account for emergency reserves, and sends the other $12,000 to his mortgage company, in addition to his normal mortgage payment. John now deposits his paycheck into the LOC and writes checks from the LOC to cover his bills. Each month the extra $1,000 reduces his LOC balance by $1,000, and at the end of 12 months the balance is $0. John then repeats this entire process until his mortgage is completely paid off.

Note: The larger the dollar amount of your excess cash flow, the faster you can transfer lump sums to pay off your mortgage and reduce your LOC balance. This is how you can use debt to pay off debt and make it work to your advantage. For example, if your excess cash flow is large enough, it is feasible that you could end up using a 10% LOC to pay off a 6% mortgage and still cut years off your loan.

Conclusion of Cash Flow Maximizer Strategy

To make the loan repayment process work, you need to have:

- Financial discipline and
- Positive monthly cash flow that you can apply consistently to your debt

If you do not consistently have extra cash flow, then you need to buckle down, create a budget to cut costs, then be responsible and follow through to achieve your final goal. When you own your home free and clear in a few years, or you've paid off all your credit cards, or added thousands of dollars to your retirement, you will be happy you made the extra effort.

The real danger is that you can be tempted to increase your credit card spending, or even worse, spend the money that you have reserved in your LOC for emergencies to take a vacation or buy a new TV. You need to avoid this temptation, or you'll end up defeating the entire purpose of cash flow maximization. In fact, you could put yourself into deeper debt that would be almost impossible to recover from.

Using an inexpensive money management software program such as Quicken could give you the financial discipline to avoid some of these temptations. This software can make it much easier to identify money that is being wasted and can now be saved.

Financial discipline and a positive cash flow are the keys to making the loan repayment process successful.

CHAPTER 4

PAYING FOR COLLEGE IN A TAX-EFFICIENT MANNER

EDUCATION TAX INCENTIVES

American Opportunity Tax Credit (for Undergraduate Students)

The American Opportunity Credit (AOC) is a nonrefundable credit against an individual's federal income tax liability.

Calculation of Credit

The AOC is calculated by taking 100% of the first $2,000 of "qualified tuition and related expenses" plus 25% of the excess of these expenses up to a $2,000 limit.

Example: If the qualified expenses of an individual student were $4,500, the AOC would be $2,500 (100% × $2,000 + 25% × $2,000). If the expenses were only

$2,200, the AOC would be $2,050 (100% × $2,000 + 25% × $200).

Maximum Credit Allowed

The maximum AOC allowed per student is $2,500 per year. The credit can be claimed for each student on the parents' tax return.

For example, if there are two "eligible students" who have qualified expenses, a maximum AOC of $5,000 (2 students × $2,500) can be claimed.

Credit Phaseout

The AOC is phased out when the taxpayer reaches certain levels of "modified adjusted gross income." The credit is ratably phased out for modified adjusted gross income (AGI) of between $80,000 and $90,000 for single and head-of-household taxpayers and between $160,000 and $180,000 for married taxpayers for the year 2019.

Example: A married taxpayer with $170,000 in modified AGI would have a maximum AOC of $1,250 per eligible student.

Qualified Expenses

The AOC is only available for certain qualified expenses for undergraduate courses at "eligible educational institutions." Qualified expenses are tuition and related fees at these eligible educational institutions; they do not include books, room and board, personal transportation or living expenses, activity fees, or insurance. The qualified expenses have to actually be paid during the academic period or, if paid in a prior tax year, the academic period must begin within the first 3 months of the next year.

The qualified expenses are reduced by tax-free grants or scholarships, employer-provided educational assistance, veteran's education benefits, tax-free withdrawals from a Qualified Tuition Plan or Coverdell Education Savings Account, and qualified expenses deducted elsewhere on the tax return.

Only out-of-pocket qualified expenses are used to calculate the AOC. The expenses may be paid by the student, the parents of the student, or a third party, such as a grandparent, for the student. The expenses can be paid, with no reduction in qualified expenses, by loans, savings, savings from a qualified tuition program, gifts, bequests, devises, or inheritances.

Note: Loan repayments for qualified expenses do not count as qualified expenses in calculating the AOC.

Example: Harry has enrolled in a postsecondary vocational program in September of 2018 that requires $1,500 for tuition. Harry's second semester of this program begins February 3, 2019, and again requires about $1,500 for tuition, due by January 31, 2019. To maximize the 2018 AOC, Harry's parents are permitted to prepay tuition in December of 2018 for the academic period beginning in February 2019. Accordingly, Harry's parents should prepay $1,250 of tuition in December of 2018 to qualify for the full $2,500 AOC in their 2018 Form 1040.

If a third party, defined as someone other than the taxpayer, taxpayer's spouse, or a claimed dependent, makes a payment directly to the educational institution toward the tuition fee, the tuition is treated as paid by the student for purposes of the credits.

Eligible Students

The student must be enrolled in a degree, certificate, or other program leading to a recognized educational credential at an eligible educational institution; this includes an approved program of study abroad. The student must be enrolled on at least a half-time basis, which is usually six credits.

To be eligible for the AOC, the student must not have been convicted of a federal or state drug felony offense consisting of the possession or distribution of a controlled substance.

Lifetime Learning Credit

The lifetime learning credit (LLC) is a nonrefundable credit against the individual's federal income tax liability.

Calculation of Credit

The LLC is calculated by taking 20% of up to a maximum of $10,000 in "qualified tuition and related expenses." The limit for the LLC is $2,000 per taxpayer tax return.

Example: If a family has a combined total of $12,000 in qualified tuition expenses for all the exemptions claimed on the tax return, the LLC for the tax return would be $2,000, 20% × $10,000 maximum qualified expenses. If the same family had combined total expenses of only $8,000, the LLC would be $1,600, 20% × $8,000.

Maximum Credit Allowed

The maximum LLC allowed is $2,000 per taxpayer return, not per eligible student. The qualified expenses for all eligible students can be combined to reach the maximum credit of $2,000.

Example: If there are two eligible students and each has qualified expense of $10,000, the maximum LLC that could be claimed is $2,000 per that taxpayer return.

Credit Phaseout

The LLC is phased out when the taxpayer reaches certain levels:

- $57,000 to $67,000, for single or head of household.

- $114,000 to $134,000 for married taxpayers of the modified AGI.

- A married taxpayer, with $124,000 modified AGI, would have a maximum LLC of $1,000.

▶ **PLANNING TIP 1**

As a tax planning strategy, families who have a modified AGI in excess of the phaseout levels (single or head of household, $67,000, or married taxpayers, $134,000) may want to give up the student as a tax exemption. The student can then claim the LLC, provided the student's modified AGI is also not above the phaseout limits.

> ▶ **PLANNING TIP 2**
>
> Another tax planning strategy to consider for families with two students in college at the same time is for the parents to give up one of the students as a tax exemption. This student can then claim the LLC for the expenses on his or her tax return, provided the student's modified AGI is not above the phaseout limits. In addition, the other student's qualified expenses could be claimed for the LLC on the parents' tax return, provided the parents' modified AGI is not above the phaseout limits. The overall result of this strategy would be that two LLCs, instead of only one LLC, could be claimed by this family on the two separate taxpayer returns.

Qualified Expenses

The LLC is available for certain qualified expenses for undergraduate, graduate, or professional degree courses at eligible educational institutions. Qualified expenses are the same as for the AOC and for tuition and related fees at these eligible educational institutions, but they do not include books, room and board, personal transportation or living expenses, activity fees, or insurance. The qualified expenses have to actually be paid during the academic period or, if paid in a prior tax year, the academic period must begin within the first 3 months of the next year.

The qualified expenses are reduced by tax-free grants or scholarships, employer-provided educational assistance, veterans' education benefits, tax-free withdrawals from a Qualified Tuition Plan or Coverdell Education

Savings Account, and qualified expenses deducted elsewhere on the tax return.

Only out-of-pocket qualified expenses are used to calculate the LLC. The expenses may be paid by the student, the parents of the student, or a third party, such as a grandparent, for the student. The expenses can be paid, with no reduction in qualified expenses, by loans, savings, savings from a qualified tuition program, gifts, bequests, devises, or inheritances.

Note: Loan repayments for qualified expenses do not count as qualified expenses in calculating the LLC.

If a third party, defined as someone other than the taxpayer, taxpayer's spouse, or a claimed dependent, makes a payment directly to the educational institution toward the tuition fee, the tuition is treated as paid by the student for purposes of the credits.

Eligible Students

- There is no limit to the number of years in which an eligible student may claim the LLC. The student must be the taxpayer, the taxpayer's spouse, or a dependent of the taxpayer.

- The student may be enrolled less than half-time and still qualify for the LLC.

- The courses, at eligible educational institutions, taken by the student are allowed to be taken to acquire or improve job skills.

- The student convicted of a federal or state drug felony can qualify for the LLC.

Student Loan Interest Deduction

A tax deduction is allowed for interest paid on qualified student loans. The taxpayer does not have to itemize deductions to claim this deduction. The loans do not have to be federal interest-subsidized loans. Any type of loan that is used to pay college costs qualifies for this interest deduction. For example, a loan taken from your life insurance policy that is used to pay for college would qualify.

Calculation of the Interest Deduction

The interest deduction is calculated by taking 100% of any interest due and paid on a qualified student loan.

Maximum Interest Deduction Allowed

The maximum interest deduction allowed is $2,500 per year.

Interest Deduction Phaseout

The deduction for student loan interest is phased out when the taxpayer reaches certain levels of modified AGI. The AGI phaseout range for the student loan interest deduction is $65,000 to $80,000 for single taxpayers and $135,000 to $165,000 for married taxpayers filing jointly.

Qualified Expenses

The student loan interest deduction is only available for qualified expenses for undergraduate or graduate courses. The loan must have been used to pay the cost of attendance at an eligible educational institution.

These expenses include tuition, fees, room and board, supplies, equipment, transportation, and related personal expenses.

Note: Qualified expenses for the interest deduction include more items than are allowed for the AOC or Lifetime Learning Tax Credit.

Qualified expenses do not include expenses paid by an intrafamily loan. Also, qualified expenses do not include expenses paid with a loan from a qualified employer retirement plan.

Eligible Students

To be eligible for the interest deduction, the student must be enrolled, on at least a half-time basis, in a program leading to a degree, certificate, or other recognized educational credential. The student must be the taxpayer, the taxpayer's spouse, or a dependent of the taxpayer at the time the loans were received. No deduction is allowed for an individual who is claimed as a dependent on another taxpayer's tax return.

Qualified Education Loan

The loan must have been incurred solely to pay qualified higher education expenses at an eligible institution. The higher education expenses must be paid or incurred within a reasonable period of time before or after the debt originates.

Financial Aid Consequences

The student loan interest deduction increases the financial aid eligibility of any student who is currently enrolled in college. As the interest deduction lowers the income of the parents or student, it could increase the financial aid eligibility by the amount of the interest deduction times the parents' financial aid income assessment rate of 22% to 47%, or the student's financial aid income assessment rate of 50%.

The Education Assistance Program

Several thousand companies offer tuition assistance programs as a fringe benefit for employees who want to further their college studies. The tax treatment of these Employer Educational Assistance Programs (IRS Section 127) can be tax deductible to the employer and also tax-free, up to $5,250 per year, to the employee. This benefit is also available for students who are enrolled in graduate-level studies.

Employers are not required to offer educational assistance to employees. However, with increased technology in the workplace, the continuing education of employees is necessary to ensure that the employer stays competitive in the marketplace. Many employers recognize this and choose to offer educational assistance benefits.

Example of the Educational Assistance Program Strategy:

Tom is a self-employed business owner whose 21-year-old son will be a junior in college this year. As Tom's son is employed in his business during the summer months, Tom can deduct tuition and fees incurred during the next two years of school. If Tom's son needs a fifth year to graduate, he can deduct tuition and fees for that year also. If his son decides to attend graduate school, Tom can deduct the graduate school tuition and fees also (up to $5,250 per year).

Tom currently pays 25% in federal taxes, 6% in state taxes and 15.3% in self-employment taxes, for a total tax rate of 46.3%. Assuming Tom's son will graduate in two years (and incurs at least $5,250 in tuition costs each year), Tom can now deduct $5,250 each year for those two years, which will result in a tax savings of $2,431 each year ($5,250 × 46.3% = $2,431).

Penalty-Free IRA Withdrawals

Penalty-free withdrawals from regular IRAs can be made to pay for undergraduate or graduate qualified higher education expenses for the taxpayer, the taxpayer's spouse, or the child or grandchild of the taxpayer or taxpayer's spouse at an eligible educational institution. The taxpayer will owe federal income tax on the amount withdrawn, but will not be subject to the 10% early withdrawal penalty imposed when amounts are withdrawn from an IRA before the taxpayer reaches the age of 59½.

Qualified Expenses

The penalty-free IRA withdrawal is only available if the withdrawal is used to pay for qualified education expenses. Qualified education expenses include tuition, fees, books, supplies, and equipment. Room and board are also included if the student is enrolled on at least a half-time basis. These education expenses must be reduced by any tax-free scholarships or grants, qualified U.S. Series EE bonds, veterans' education benefits, and other tax-free educational benefits.

Eligible Students

To be eligible for the penalty-free IRA distribution, the student must be the taxpayer or the taxpayer's spouse, and attend an eligible educational institution.

SAVING AND PAYING FOR FUTURE COLLEGE COSTS IN A TAX-ADVANTAGED MANNER

Introduction to Tax Capacity

When planning for college, you must be aware of the many income tax strategies available to increase the amount of family funds for future college costs. Although these strategies may not produce a direct college benefit, like a grant or scholarship, they may lead to tax benefits to your family as a whole, and thereby increase the amount of family funds available to pay for college. To gain the maximum effect of these strategies, you must utilize the education tax incentives discussed in the previous section. The combination of the income tax strategies and education tax incentives described in this module will enable you to save and/or pay for college in a tax-efficient manner.

Because some families are not eligible for financial aid, they are not penalized by a loss of financial aid for shifting income and assets to their children.

Therefore, they should take full advantage of a child's lower tax bracket by shifting income and assets to the child. Accordingly, a key strategy is to focus on the benefits of the tax system. This will be driven by taking advantage of opportunities in the child's tax return (i.e., the child's lower tax bracket) not available to the parent or grandparent. *Tax capacity* is the amount of income that can be shifted to a child, and have the child still be taxed in a lower tax bracket than the parents' tax bracket.

Tax Capacity Time Frames

A child's tax capacity can be divided into two time frames:

1. Birth through age 18 and dependent students through age 23, the "kiddie tax" year

2. Age 24 and above

To properly plan the use of your child's tax return, you must understand your child's tax capacity and tax opportunities for each of these time frames.

Birth Through Age 23: Kiddie Tax Years

During the period from birth through age 23, a child's tax capacity is limited by the kiddie tax. The liddie tax is applied to the investment income, such as interest, dividends, or rental income, of a child under age 24 that exceeds $2,100. The investment income in excess of $2,100 is taxed at the high trust tax rates, rather than the child's lower rates. Earned income, such as wages, is not subject to the kiddie tax at any age.

Example: A 22-year-old child has interest income of $1,950. The kiddie tax does not apply because investment income does not exceed $2,100.

As the kiddie tax applies only to unearned income of a child under 23 years of age, one option for avoiding the kiddie tax is to invest the child's assets in investments that produce tax-exempt income or defer the income until after the child reaches age 24. Efficient use of the child's tax capacity, however, would suggest that the child can absorb at least $2,100 of unearned income, tax-free annually.

Age 24 and Older

When a child reaches age 24, the kiddie tax rules no longer apply. Therefore, you should be aware of your child's increased tax capacity. This increased tax capacity should be factored into the college-funding plan.

This amount of income can be shifted to the child from a parent or grandparent and be sheltered from the parents' higher income tax bracket.

If the child has a tax liability, the tax liability can then be offset by the American Opportunity Credit or LLC. These credits can only be claimed if the child is not a tax dependent of the parents. Note that the child does not have to provide more than half of his or her financial support to claim these tax credits.

Income-Shifting Strategies

Income shifting from parents or grandparents, to children or grandchildren, to take advantage of the child's tax capacity is accomplished by putting income-producing assets in the children's or grandchildren's name. The related income generated by these assets is taxed at the child's lower income tax rates, and thus, the family receives a tax benefit. This tax benefit or "tax scholarship" will help increase the amount of funds available for college. In addition to the income tax savings, there may also be considerable estate tax savings earned by shifting the asset to a child or grandchild. Several income-shifting techniques are discussed in this section.

Methods of Income Shifting

Parents can shift assets and the resulting income in one of many ways. Five of the most common ways to shift income are:

- Gifting appreciated assets during college years
- Compensating the child
- Giving assets that will earn and grow
- Gift/sale and leaseback
- Gifts of business interest

Shifting by Gifting Appreciated Assets During College Years

Gifts of appreciated assets to the child from the parents may be an effective method of shifting income to the child. If the gift is not made until the child needs the money for college, the parent can keep control of the asset until it is needed for college.

Shifting Income by Compensating the Child

Parents with businesses or rentals who can pay compensation to the child achieve tax benefits that can be used to pay part of the college cost.

In addition to the tax saving benefits of hiring a child, the child would be eligible to save for college, because of the earned income, by purchasing either Roth or regular IRAs. The tax-deferred growth over a long term can result in very substantial accumulations when the child reaches college age. The Roth IRA may be the best type of IRA to use because the original contributions may be withdrawn tax and penalty-free for college expenses. If the child has other unearned income that is creating income tax, a traditional IRA should be considered.

Shifting by Giving Assets that Earn and Grow in Precollege Years

For parents with no appreciated assets or family compensation opportunities, an alternative strategy is to shift assets to the child as early as possible by annual gifts, so that the growth and earnings on the investments are taxed at the child's rates rather than parental rates.

In general, the strategy should be to defer all investment income to college years to take advantage of the education tax credits.

Use of a custodial account is a common vehicle to hold the assets shifted to a child in precollege years. These accounts are simple and inexpensive to establish. The custodian of the account is responsible to see that the account assets are spent for the benefit of the child.

This method of income shifting could be utilized by parents who want to keep the control of the asset out of the child's hands until the child is 18 or 21 years of age. Parents can reduce their estate and provide a college fund for their child by using a custodial account. If the parents are giving a small or moderate amount of assets to their child and do not want the high administrative costs associated with trusts, a custodial account should be considered.

▶ **PLANNING TIP 3**

Nonqualified stock options and incentive stock options (ISOs) can be used to shift income to children at capital gain rates. By making lifetime gifts of nonqualified stock options before the market value has appreciated, an employee may remove a potential high-growth asset from an estate, at a low gift tax value. By permitting an employee to transfer nonqualified stock options to children or grandchildren, a company may confer a substantial benefit without additional compensation expense and the employee will have an appreciated asset to gift to his children. The children will sell the stock to pay for college and will be taxed at the child's lower capital gain rates.

▶ **PLANNING TIP 4**

If you are aware of an investment that has appreciation potential, instead of purchasing the investment, you could direct your child to make the investment. If necessary, sufficient cash or other assets can be given to your child so that he or she can make the purchase.

Gift/Sale and Leaseback

Taxpayers who own a business can save taxes by shifting income to their children. One good income-shifting method is to lease business property from them. The property can be an office building, a warehouse, computer or telephone equipment, cars, trucks, or any office equipment. There are two basic ways that you can provide your children with the resources to acquire the property that your business will lease.

1. Gift and leaseback: This arrangement works when you have direct (personal) ownership of some property that is being used by your business. By using a gift and leaseback arrangement, you can gift the property to a child or to a trust (or limited partnership) for all of your children. Your business would then enter into a rental or lease agreement with the child (guardian) or trust.

2. Sale and leaseback: This is a more common arrangement when your corporation owns the property. Corporations can't make nontaxable gifts, so a transfer of property by a corporation may be through a sale of the property. To make a gift to a child, your corporation would first have to make a taxable distribution of the property to you. In a sale and leaseback arrangement, the corporation would sell the property to a child (trust) and then lease the property back from the child (trust).

Sales and leaseback transactions are not subject to gift taxes as long as the sale is a bona fide transaction and the sales price is equal to the fair market value of the related property. A gift and leaseback of the property would require a gift tax return if the amount is more than $15,000 ($30,000 for joint gifts).

Example of the Gift/Sale and Leaseback Strategy
Tom is a self-employed business owner and he and his wife gifted a $26,000 car (within the IRS gift guidelines) to their 20-year-old son, who is an employee of the business. The car was five years old and fully depreciated, so Tom was no longer able to take tax deductions for the vehicle. Tom then completed an agreement with his son to lease the car back to Tom's company for $400 per month for four years.

Tom currently pays 25% in federal taxes, 6% in state taxes, and 15.3% in self-employment taxes, for a total tax rate of 46.3%. As the $26,000 car was fully depreciated, Tom could no longer deduct the car from his business. However, using the gift and leaseback strategy, Tom can now deduct the lease payments of $4,800 per year ($400 × 12 months) from his business profit. As a result, he will save $2,222 in taxes ($400/month × 12 = $4,800 × 46.3%) each year for the next four years.

Gifts of Business Interest

There are other income-shifting techniques that may be used by the parents to shift income to their child. The

following techniques can be used to shift income to a
child:

1. Gifts of S corporation stock to the child to shift
   part of the earnings to the child
2. Gifts of limited liability company interests to
   shift part of the earnings to the child
3. Gifts of family limited partnership interests to
   shift part of the earnings to the child

CHAPTER 5

CASE STUDIES

REGISTERED NURSE WITH TWO CHILDREN; HUSBAND IS A BUSINESS OWNER

Donna Reynolds is a full-time registered nurse (RN) currently employed at a medical clinic, earning $80,000 per year. Joe Reynolds owns a real estate business with earnings averaging about $70,000 per year. They have two children, ages 9 and 12.

Donna wants to obtain her MSN degree, which will not only increase her future salary but also provide her with new career opportunities, and the extra earnings will help defray the costs of upcoming college expenses for their two children.

To complete the MSN program in 24 months, Donna will have to quit her job and attend school full-time. The advanced degree program will cost $100,000. The family goals are:

(*continued*)

- Pay for the immediate cost of Donna's advanced nursing degree.

- Create enough cash flow to retain the family's current lifestyle.

Note: The "true cost" of the advanced nursing degree is the $100,000 college cost plus the loss of income of $160,000 over the 24-month period ($80,000/year wage × 2) for a total "true cost" of $260,000.

Financial Information

- **Assets:**
  - Home value: $450,000
  - Mom's 401(k) value: $84,000 ($600/month contribution)
  - Dad's Roth IRA value: $55,000 ($500/month contribution)
  - Checking/savings: $18,000
  - Vehicles (2) value: $42,000
- **Debt:**
  - Home mortgage: $215,000 ($1,300/month payment)
  - Vehicle debt: $35,000 ($900/month payment)
  - Installment debt: $6,000 ($200/month payment)

- Credit card debt: $7,000 ($500/month payment)
- Federal income taxes paid is approximately $25,000 per year
- Health insurance premiums paid is approximately $18,000 per year
- Living expenses are approximately $50,000 per year

- **Family goals:**
  - Pay for the immediate cost of Mom's advanced nursing degree.
  - Create enough cash flow to keep the family's current lifestyle.

Table 5.1 shows the family's initial financial situation taken from the preceding financial information. Table 5.2 shows their projected financial situation after implementing some financial strategies.

Columns A and B contain the family's initial financial situation.

- The initial net cash flow for the family of $699 is at the bottom of Column B.

- The net cash flow is calculated by subtracting "Total Expenses" ($7,800), "Total Asset Contributions" ($1,100), and "Total Liabilities Payments" ($2,900) from "Total Income" ($12,499).

Columns C and D contain the adjustments to the initial financial situation.

TABLE 5.1 Family's Initial Financial Situation

	A		B	
	INITIAL ASSET/ LIABILITY		INITIAL MONTHLY CONT/PAYMENT	
Income				
W-2 (Gross)			$	6,666
Interest/Dividends				
Business			$	5,833
Rent				
Other				
Total Income	$	–	$	12,499
Expenses				
Health Insurance			$	1,500
Living Expenses			$	4,200
College			$	–
Income Taxes			$	2,100
Total Expenses	$	–	$	7,800
Assets				
Retirement	$	139,000	$	1,100
Residence	$	450,000		
Vehicles	$	42,000		
Other	$	18,000		
Total Assets	$	649,000	$	1,100
Liabilities				
Home Mortgage	$	215,000	$	1,300
Vehicle	$	35,000	$	900
Installment	$	6,000	$	200
Credit Card	$	7,000	$	500
Other				
Total Liabilities	$	263,000	$	2,900
Net Assets & Liabilities	$	386,000	$	699

TABLE 5.2 Family's Projected Financial Situation

	A	B	C	D	E	F
	INITIAL ASSET/ LIABILITY	INITIAL MONTHLY CONT/PAYMENT	MONTHLY CONT/PAYMENT ADJUSTMENT	ASSET/ LIABILITY ADJUSTMENT	REVISED ASSET/ LIABILITY	REVISED MONTHLY CONT/ PAYMENT
Income						
W-2 (Gross)		$ 6,666	$ (1) (6,666)			$ –
Interest/ Dividends						$ –
Business		$ 5,833	$ –			$ 5,833
Retirement Withdrawal			$ (6) 1,300			$ 1,300
Other		$ –	$ (2) 3,750			$ 3,750
Total Income	$ –	$ 12,499	$ (1,616)	$ –	$ –	$ 10,883
Expenses Health Insurance		$ 1,500	$ (3) (1,250)			$ 250
Living Expenses		$ 4,200				$ 4,200
College		$ –	$ (4) 3,750			$ 3,750
Income Taxes		$ 2,100	$ (5) (1,600)			$ 500
Total Expenses	$ –	$ 7,800	$ 900	$ –	$ –	$ 8,700

(continued)

TABLE 5.2 Family's Projected Financial Situation (continued)

	A INITIAL ASSET/ LIABILITY	B INITIAL MONTHLY CONT/PAYMENT	C MONTHLY CONT/PAYMENT ADJUSTMENT	D ASSET/ LIABILITY ADJUSTMENT	E REVISED ASSET/ LIABILITY	F REVISED MONTHLY CONT/ PAYMENT
Assets Retirement	$ 139,000	$ 1,100	$ (6) (1,100)	$ –	$ 139,000	$ –
Residence	$ 450,000	$ –	$ –	$ –	$ 450,000	$ –
Vehicles	$ 42,000	$ –	$ –	$ –	$ 42,000	$ –
Other	$ 18,000	$ –	$ –	$ –	$ 18,000	$ –
Total Assets	**$ 649,000**	**$ 1,100**	**$ (1,100)**	**$ –**	**$ 649,000**	**$ –**
Liabilities						
Home Mortgage	$ 215,000	$ 1,300	$ (7) 150	$ 48,000	$ 263,000	$ 1,450
Vehicle	$ 35,000	$ 900	$ (8) (900)	$ (35,000)	$ –	$ –
Installment	$ 6,000	$ 200	$ (9) (200)	$ (6,000)	$ –	$ –
Credit Card	$ 7,000	$ 500	$ (10) (500)	$ (7,000)	$ –	$ –
Other		$ 635	$ (11) 635	$ 90,000	$ 90,000	$ 635
Total Liabilities	**$ 263,000**	**$ 2,900**	**$ (815)**	**$ 90,000**	**$ 353,000**	**$ 2,085**
Net Assets & Cash Flow	**$ 386,000**	**$ 699**	**$ (601)**	**$ (90,000)**	**$ 296,000**	**$ 98**

1. As Donna has to quit her job, the initial monthly W-2 income of $6,666 will be reduced by $6,666.

2. It is anticipated that Donna will receive monthly student loan proceeds of $3,750.

3. As the family's income has been reduced by $80,000, they will receive tax subsidies to pay for their health insurance and reduce their monthly health insurance cost by $1,250 per month.

4. Graduate school expenses of $3,750 per month will be incurred over a 24-month period.

5. As the family's income will be reduced by $80,000, their income taxes will be reduced by $1,600 per month.

6. The family plans to discontinue their $1,100 monthly retirement account contributions during the college years.

7. Donna also wants to take a $1,300-per-month loan from her retirement account during college years. The combination of these two strategies will create an additional $1,300 of positive cash flow during college years. Once Donna graduates and starts earning again, they will make up for the reduced retirement contributions.

8. The family plans to consolidate their vehicle, installment, and credit card debts into a second mortgage on their home. This will increase their monthly home payments by $150 per month.

9. As these debts were consolidated into a second mortgage on the home, the monthly payments on these debts are reduced to zero.

10. The monthly loan payment of $635 on Donna's student loan debt of $90,000 is added to the monthly debt payments.

Columns E and F contain the revised financial situation.

- The revised net cash flow for the family ($98) is at the bottom of Column F.

- The revised net cash flow is calculated by subtracting revised "Total Expenses" ($8,700), total revised asset contributions ($1,300), and revised "Total Liabilities" ($2,085) from revised "Total Income" ($9,583).

Bottom Line

Even with Donna's income reduction of $80,000 per year, $100,000 of graduate school expenses were paid while still maintaining a positive cash flow and their current lifestyle. This was accomplished by implementing some debt consolidation strategies and suspending retirement plan contributions during the college period.

CASE STUDY #2

GRAD STUDENT FROM A HIGH-INCOME FAMILY; PARENTS SUPPORTING A GRAD STUDENT AND AN UNDERGRADUATE STUDENT SIMULTANEOUSLY

Liz and Brian Drake are a high-income family with their two children in college. Brian earns approximately $20,000 per month as a senior vice president at a medical supply company. Liz is a pharmaceutical sales rep earning $12,000 per month. They also receive $500 per month in dividends from an investment.

Their 22-year-old daughter, Elena, is pursuing her MSN degree at a public university that costs $45,000 per year. Her 18-year-old brother, Mark, is a freshman student at a public university costing $25,000 per year. The parents expect to incur $100,000 in costs for Mark attending undergraduate school, and they anticipate the debt for Elena's graduate school will be about $100,000. They sought a college financial planner for a strategic plan to pay the cost of college for their children.

The family strategy:

1. Pay for the cost of undergraduate school by selling $100,000 of stock options without paying income tax on the gain

2. Create enough cash flow by reducing income taxes to make the loan payments on the loans of $100,000 taken out to pay for graduate school.

Financial Information

- **Assets:**
  - Home value: $650,000
  - Liz's (the mother) 401(k) value: $184,000 ($700/month contribution)
  - Brian's (the father) 401(k) value: $248,000 ($800/month contribution)
  - Checking/Savings: $18,000
  - Stock options value: $142,000
  - Vehicles (2) value: $52,000
- **Debt:**
  - Home mortgage: $415,000 ($2,100/month payment)
  - Vehicle debt: $35,000 ($900/month payment)
  - Installment debt: $6,000 ($200/month payment)
  - Credit card debt: $7,000 ($500/month payment)
  - Federal income taxes paid are approximately $7,900 per month
  - Living expenses are approximately $13,000 per month

Tables 5.3 and 5.4 show the family's initial financial situation taken from the preceding financial information and their projected financial situation after implementing some financial strategies.

TABLE 5.3 Family's Initial Financial Situation

	A	B
	INITIAL ASSET/ LIABILITY	**INITIAL MONTHLY CONT/PAYMENT**
Income		
W-2 (Gross)		$ 32,000
Interest/Dividends		$ 500
Business		$ –
Rent		$ –
Other		$ –
Total Income	$ –	$ **32,500**
Expenses		
Health Insurance		$ –
Living Expenses		$ 13,000
College		$ –
Income Taxes		$ 7,900
Total Expenses	$ –	$ **20,900**
Assets		
Retirement	$ 432,000	$ 1,500
Investments	$ 142,000	$ –
Business	$ –	$ –
Residence	$ 650,000	$ –
Vehicles	$ 52,000	$ –
Other	$ 18,000	$ –
Total Assets	$ **1,294,000**	$ **1,500**
Liabilities		
Home Mortgage	$ 415,000	$ 2,100
Vehicles	$ 35,000	$ 900
Installment	$ 6,000	$ 200
Credit Card	$ 7,000	$ 500
Other	$ 100,000	$ 670
Total Liabilities	$ **563,000**	$ **4,370**
Net Assets & Cash Flow	$ **731,000**	$ **5,730**

TABLE 5.4 Family's Projected Financial Situation

	A INITIAL ASSET/ LIABILITY	B INITIAL MONTHLY CONT/PAYMENT	C MONTHLY CONT/PAYMENT ADJUSTMENT		D ASSET/ LIABILITY ADJUSTMENT	E REVISED ASSET/ LIABILITY	F REVISED MONTHLY CONT/PAYMENT
Income							
W-2 (Gross)		$ 32,000	$	–			$ 32,000
Interest/ Dividends		$ 500					$ 500
Business		$ –	$	–			$ –
Rent		$ –	$	–			$ –
Other		$ –	$	–			$ –
Total Income	$ –	$ 32,500	$	–	$ –	$ –	$ 32,500
Expenses Health Insurance		$ –	$ (1)	580			$ 580
Living Expenses		$ 13,000	$	–			$ 13,000
College		$ –	$	–			$ –
Income Taxes		$ 7,900	$ (2)	(1,035)			$ 6,865
Total Expenses	$ –	$ 20,900	$	(455)	$ –	$ –	$ 20,445

Assets						
Retirement	$ 432,000	$ 1,500	$ (3) 2,666	$ –	$ 432,000	$ 4,166
Investments	$ 142,000	$ –	$ –	$ (100,000)	$ 42,000	$ –
Business	$ –	$ –		$ –	$ –	$ –
Residence	$ 650,000	$ –	$ –	$ –	$ 650,000	$ –
Vehicles	$ 52,000	$ –	$ –	$ –	$ 52,000	$ –
Other	$ 18,000	$ –	$ –	$ –	$ 18,000	$ –
Total Assets	**$ 1,294,000**	**$ 1,500**	**$ 2,666**	**$ (100,000)**	**$ 1,194,000**	**$ 4,166**
Liabilities						
Home Mortgage	$ 415,000	$ 2,100	$ –	$ –	$ 415,000	$ 2,100
Vehicle	$ 35,000	$ 900	$ –	$ –	$ 35,000	$ 900
Installment	$ 6,000	$ 200	$ –	$ –	$ 6,000	$ 200
Credit Card	$ 7,000	$ 500	$ –		$ 7,000	$ 500
Other	$ 100,000	$ 670			$ 100,000	$ 670
Total Liabilities	**$ 563,000**	**$ 4,370**	**$ –**	**$ –**	**$ 563,000**	**$ 4,370**
Net Assets & Cash Flow	**$ 731,000**	**$ 5,730**	**$ (2,211)**	**$ (100,000)**	**$ 631,000**	**$ 3,519**

Columns A and B of Tables 5.3 and 5.4 contain the family's initial financial situation.

The initial net cash flow for the family of $5,730 is at the bottom of Column B.

The net cash flow is calculated by subtracting "Total Expenses" ($20,900), "Total Asset Contributions" ($1,500), and "Total Liabilities Payments" ($4,370) from "Total Income" ($32,500).

Columns C and D of Table 5.4 contain the adjustments to the initial financial situation.

Adjustments to the initial financial situation:

1. The parents plan to open a Health Savings Account (HSA) and contribute $580 per month. This will lower their income taxes by $185 per month.

2. The parents' income taxes will decrease by $1,035 per month because of their contributions to the HSA ($185/month) and the increased contributions to their 401(k)s ($850/month).

3. The parents plan to increase their 401(k) contributions by $2,666 per month for a total of $4,166 per month. This will lower their income taxes by $850 per month.

Columns E and F contain the revised financial situation.

The revised net cash flow for the family of $3,519 is at the bottom of Column F.

The revised net cash flow is calculated by subtracting "Revised Total Expenses" ($20,455), "Total Revised Asset Contributions" ($4,166), and "Total Revised

Liabilities Payments" ($4,370) from "Total Revised Income" ($32,500).

Bottom Line

The parents will increase their retirement account, deduct their medical costs through the HSA, make the loan payments for graduate school, and pay for undergraduate school using tax-free stock options, while maintaining a positive cash flow and their current lifestyle.

CASE STUDY #3

FAMILY WITH AN S CORPORATION BUSINESS SUPPORTING THREE CHILDREN

Grace and David Burke own a business operated as an S corporation which provides them with a net income of $12,500 per month. They also receive $1,500 from rental income each month. Grace and David have three children ages 22, 18, and 16.

The 16-year-old attends a private high school costing $21,000 per year. The 18-year-old is a freshman at a public university that costs $30,000 per year. The 22-year-old student is enrolled in a two-year nursing master's program.

The family goals are:

- Pay for the cost of K-to-12 private school and undergraduate school using tax savings.

- Create enough cash flow by reducing income taxes to make the loan payments on the loans taken out to pay for graduate school.

Financial Information

- **Assets:**
  - Home value: $550,000
  - Dad's IRA value: $148,000 ($500/month contribution)
  - Checking/Savings: $18,000
  - Business value: $742,000
  - Vehicles (2) value: $52,000

■ **Debt:**

▪ Home mortgage: $215,000 ($1,100/month payment)

▪ Vehicle debt: $35,000 ($900/month payment)

▪ Installment debt: $6,000 ($200/month payment)

▪ Credit card debt: $7,000 ($500/month payment)

▪ Federal income taxes paid are approximately $1,900 per month

▪ Living expenses are approximately $6,000 per month

▪ Healthcare insurance expenses are approximately $2,700 per month

Tables 5.5 and 5.6 show the family's initial financial situation taken from the preceding financial information and their projected financial situation after implementing some financial strategies.

Columns A and B contain the family's initial financial situation.

■ The initial net cash flow for the family of negative $3,800 is at the bottom of Column B.

The net cash flow is calculated by subtracting "Total Expenses" ($14,600), "Total Asset Contributions" ($500), and "Total Liabilities Payments" ($2,700) from "Total Income" ($14,000).

TABLE 5.5 Family's Initial Financial Situation

	A		B	
	INITIAL ASSET/ LIABILITY		**INITIAL MONTHLY CONT/PAYMENT**	
Income				
W-2 (Gross)			$	12,500
Interest/Dividends			$	–
Business			$	–
Rent			$	1,500
Other			$	–
Total Income	$	–	$	**14,000**
Expenses				
Health Insurance			$	2,700
Living Expenses			$	6,000
College			$	4,000
Income Taxes			$	1,900
Total Expenses	$	–	$	**14,600**
Assets				
Retirement	$	148,000	$	500
Business	$	742,000	$	–
Residence	$	550,000	$	–
Vehicles	$	52,000	$	–
Other	$	18,000	$	–
Total Assets	$	**1,510,000**	$	**500**
Liabilities				
Home Mortgage	$	215,000	$	1,100
Vehicle	$	35,000	$	900
Installment	$	6,000	$	200
Credit Card	$	7,000	$	500
Other	$	–	$	–
Total Liabilities	$	**263,000**	$	**2,700**
Net Assets & Cash Flow	$	**1,247,000**	$	**(3,800)**

TABLE 5.6 Family's Projected Financial Situation

	INITIAL ASSET/ LIABILITY	INITIAL MONTHLY CONT/PAYMENT	MONTHLY CONT/PAYMENT ADJUSTMENT		ASSET/ LIABILITY ADJUSTMENT	REVISED ASSET/ LIABILITY	REVISED MONTHLY CONT/PAYMENT
Income							
W-2 (Gross)		$ 12,500	$	–			$ 12,500
Interest/ Dividends		$ –					$ –
Business		$ –	$	–			$ –
Rent		$ 1,500	$	–			$ 1,500
Other		$ –	$	–			$ –
Total Income	$ –	$ 14,000	$	–	$ –	$ –	$ 14,000
Expenses							
Health Insurance		$ 2,700	$ (1)	(1,800)			$ 900
Living Expenses		$ 6,000	$	–			$ 6,000
College		$ 4,000	$ (2)	(1,200)			$ 2,800
Income Taxes		$ 1,900	$ (3)	(1,450)			$ 450
Total Expenses	$ –	$ 14,600	$	(4,450)	$ –	$ –	$ 10,150

(continued)

TABLE 5.6 Family's Projected Financial Situation (continued)

	INITIAL ASSET/ LIABILITY	INITIAL MONTHLY CONT/PAYMENT	MONTHLY CONT/PAYMENT ADJUSTMENT	ASSET/ LIABILITY ADJUSTMENT	REVISED ASSET/ LIABILITY	REVISED MONTHLY CONT/PAYMENT
Assets						
Retirement	$ 148,000	$ 500	$ —	$ —	$ 148,000	$ 500
Investments	$ —	$ —	$ —	$ —	$ —	$ —
Business	$ 742,000	$ —	$ —	$ —	$ 742,000	$ —
Residence	$ 550,000	$ —	$ —	$ —	$ 550,000	$ —
Vehicles	$ 52,000	$ —	$ —	$ —	$ 52,000	$ —
Other	$ 18,000	$ —	$ —	$ —	$ 18,000	$ —
Total Assets	**$1,510,000**	**$ 500**	**$ —**	**$ —**	**$ 1,510,000**	**$ 500**
Liabilities						
Home Mortgage	$ 215,000	$ 1,100	$ —	$ —	$ 215,000	$ 1,100
Vehicle	$ 35,000	$ 900	$ —	$ —	$ 35,000	$ 900
Installment	$ 6,000	$ 200	$ —	$ —	$ 6,000	$ 200
Credit Card	$ 7,000	$ 500	$ —	$ —	$ 7,000	$ 500
Other	$ —	$ —	$ (4) 600	$ 90,000	$ 90,000	$ 600
Total Liabilities	**$ 263,000**	**$ 2,700**	**$ 600**	**$ 90,000**	**$ 353,000**	**$ 3,300**
Net Assets & Cash Flow	**$1,247,000**	**$ (3,800)**	**$ 3,850**	**$ (90,000)**	**$ 1,157,000**	**$ 50**

Columns C and D contain the adjustments to the initial financial situation.

1. Because of the income reduction strategies implemented by the parents, their health insurance premiums will be reduced by $1,800/month.

2. Because of the income reduction strategies implemented by the parents, their children's college costs will decrease by $1,200/month.

3. Because of the income reduction strategies implanted by the parents, their income taxes will decrease by $1,450/month.

4. There will be loan payments of $600/month on the $90,000 loans incurred for graduate school.

Columns E and F contain the revised financial situation.

■ The revised net cash flow of $50 for the family is at the bottom of Column F.

■ The revised net cash flow is calculated by subtracting "Revised Total Expenses" ($10,150), "Total Revised Asset Contributions" ($500), and "Total Revised Liabilities Payments" ($3,300) from "Total Revised Income" ($14,000).

Bottom Line

With the decrease in health insurance costs, college costs, and income taxes, the family will be able to pay for K to 12, undergraduate costs, and the loans incurred for graduate school if they choose. The decrease in the preceding costs was made possible because of the income/tax reduction strategies discussed in Chapter 4, "Paying for College in a Tax-Efficient Manner."

CASE STUDY #4

MSN STUDENT AND UNDERGRAD STUDENT APPEALED FOR PROFESSIONAL JUDGMENT

Julia, 24 years old, was recently accepted to attend an elite university to get her MSN, which will cost $128,000. She just completed her BSN, which her parents paid for, but they told her she was on her own for graduate school. Julia's younger brother will be a freshman in college next September at the cost of $30,000 per year. Her mother was recently laid off from her job and is currently unemployed.

Julia is an independent student for financial aid purposes. The university offered her $43,000 in grants and scholarships, but she will have to borrow $85,000 to pay the balance. She was able to get a Grad PLUS Loan for which her dad agreed to cosign.

But is there a better way for this student to pay for school? Julia's dad, Ken, has an income of $29,167 per month as an attorney. Julia has only worked during the summer months, so her earnings have only been $5,000 per year.

Julia is living at home, and as the family has two students in college, she appealed her financial aid award requesting an increase in need-based grant funds. The school agreed to offer her need-based grants, but not scholarships. Julia's brother also appealed his financial aid award based on two students in college, and his instruction reduced the family's expected family contribution, which resulted in a $1,100/month saving.

(continued)

The family strategy should be:

1. Pay for the cost of undergraduate education for son, and if they choose, they can pay for Julia's MSN degree using tax savings.

2. Create enough cash flow by reducing income taxes to make the loan payments on the loans taken out to pay for graduate school.

3. If the parents opt in to pay for graduate school, they can arrange an "intrafamily" loan, with an interest rate they both agree to, that is better than the Grad PLUS Loan rate, and Julia can repay the parents.

Financial Information

- **Assets:**
  - Home value: $800,000
  - Dad's 401K value: $375,000 ($25,000/monthly contribution)
  - Mom's 401K value: 120,000 ($0/monthly contribution)
  - Checking/Savings: $34,000
  - Vehicles (2) value: $50,000
- **Debt:**
  - Home mortgage: $300,000 ($2,400/monthly payment)
  - Vehicle debt: $18,000 ($370/monthly payment)

- Credit card debt: $9,000 ($400/monthly payment)
- Federal income taxes paid is approximately $102,000 annually or $8,500 monthly
- Living expenses are approximately $9,000 per month

Tables 5.7 and 5.8 show the family's initial financial situation taken from the preceding financial information and their projected financial situation after implementing some financial strategies.

Columns A and B contain the family's initial financial situation.

- The initial net cash flow for the family of $4,497 is at the bottom of Column B.

- The net cash flow is calculated by subtracting "Total Expenses" ($20,000), "Total Asset Contributions" ($1,500), and "Total Liabilities Payments" ($3,170) from "Total Income" ($29,167).

Columns C and D contain the adjustments to the initial financial situation.

1. Because the family will have two children in college at the same time, their son's college costs will decrease by $1,100/month.

2. Because of the income reduction strategies implemented by the parents, their income taxes will decrease by $800/month.

Columns E and F contain the revised financial situation.

TABLE 5.7 Family's Initial Financial Situation

	A	B
	INITIAL ASSET/ LIABILITY	**INITIAL MONTHLY CONT/PAYMENT**
Income		
W-2 (Gross)		$ 29,167
Interest/Dividends		$ –
Business		$ –
Rent		$ –
Other		
Total Income	$ –	$ 29,167
Expenses		
Health Insurance		$ –
Living Expenses		$ 9,000
College		$ 2,500
Income Taxes		$ 8,500
Total Expenses	$ –	$ 20,000
Assets		
Retirement	$ 495,000	$ 1,500
Business	$ –	$ –
Residence	$ 800,000	$ –
Vehicles	$ 50,000	$ –
Other	$ –	$ –
Total Assets	$ 1,345,000	$ 1,500
Liabilities		
Home Mortgage	$ 300,000	$ 2,400
Vehicle	$ 18,000	$ 370
Installment	$ –	$ –
Credit Card	$ 9,000	$ 400
Other	$ –	$ –
Total Liabilities	$ 327,000	$ 3,170
Net Assets & Cash Flow	$ 1,018,000	$ 4,497

TABLE 5.8 Family's Projected Financial Situation

A INITIAL ASSET/LIABILITY	B INITIAL MONTHLY CONT/PAYMENT		C MONTHLY CONT/PAYMENT ADJUSTMENT		D ASSET/ LIABILITY ADJUSTMENT	E REVISED ASSET/LIABILITY	F REVISED MONTHLY CONT/PAYMENT	
	$	29,167	$	–			$	29,167
	$	–					$	–
	$	–	$	–			$	–
	$	–	$	–			$	–
	$	–	$	–			$	–
$ –	$	29,167	$	–	$ –	$ –	$	29,167
	$	–					$	–
	$	9,000	$	–			$	9,000
	$	2,500	$ (1)	(1,100)			$	1,400
	$	8,500	$ (2)	(800)			$	7,700
$ –	$	20,000	$	(1,900)	$ –	$ –	$	18,100

(continued)

TABLE 5.8 Family's Projected Financial Situation (continued)

	A	B	C	D	E	F
	INITIAL ASSET/LIABILITY	INITIAL MONTHLY CONT/PAYMENT	MONTHLY CONT/PAYMENT ADJUSTMENT	ASSET/ LIABILITY ADJUSTMENT	REVISED ASSET/LIABILITY	REVISED MONTHLY CONT/PAYMENT
$	495,000	$ 1,500	$ —	$ —		$ 1,500
$	—	$ —	$ —	$ —	$ —	$ —
$	—	$ —	$ —	$ —		$ —
$	800,000	$ —	$ —	$ —		$ —
$	50,000	$ —		$ —		$ —
$	—	$ —	$ —	$ —		$ —
$	1,345,000	$ 1,500	$ —	$ —	$ —	$ 1,500
$	300,000	$ 2,400	$ —	$ —		$ 2,400
$	18,000	$ 370	$ —	$ —		370
$	—	$ —	$ —	$ —		$ —
$	9,000	$ 400	$ —	$ —		400
$	—	$ —				$ —
$	327,000	$ 3,170	$ —	$ —	$ —	$ 3,170
$	1,018,000	$ 4,497	$ 1,900	$ —	$ —	$ 6,397

- The revised net cash flow of $6,397 for the family is at the bottom of Column F.
- The revised net cash flow is calculated by subtracting "Revised Total Expenses" ($18,100), "Total Revised Asset Contributions" ($1,500), and "Total Revised Liabilities Payments" ($3,170) from the "Total Revised Income" ($29,167).

Bottom Line

The decrease in their son's college costs and income taxes will likely result in an increase in the family's cash flow by $1,900 per month. This extra cash can be used either to add to their retirement account or to pay down their debt. Due to the fact that the family had two children in college at the same time, their daughter and son appealed to their colleges for additional grants and scholarships. The nursing grad program approved Julia's appeal and awarded her an additional $18,500 in grants and scholarships. The son's college reduced the family's expected family contributions that resulted in a $1,100 per month savings.

Financial aid award appeals are done on a case-by-case basis and this example is an exception to the rules, but it can be "winnable." You can't win if you don't appeal.

CASE STUDY #5

ONE PARENT PURSUING AN ADVANCED NURSING DEGREE WITH TWO CHILDREN IN COLLEGE

Linda Cornwall is a nurse at a large hospital and wants to pursue her goal of becoming a nurse anesthetist (NA). The degree is a 36-month full-time program, which would require her to leave her current position where she makes $6,667 monthly. Her husband Barry is a sole proprietor of a landscaping business and has a net income of $6,250 per month.

Linda and Barry have a 19-year-old daughter, Gail, and a 22-year-old son, Anthony. Both children attend a public four-year in-state college and live on campus. During the summer, they work for their father's landscaping business. Gail earns $4,700 as a bookkeeper and Anthony earns $5,500 through landscaping work.

Linda and Barry sought the help of a CPA who is certified in college planning, because they didn't know how they could manage all this college debt if Linda left her job. Their family goals are:

1. Pay for the cost of undergraduate education as well as Linda's (the mother's) NA degree using tax savings.

2. Create enough cash flow by reducing income taxes to make the loan payments on the loans taken out to pay for graduate school.

Financial Information

- **Assets:**
  - Home value: $300,000
  - Barry's (Dad) IRA value: $55,000 ($500/monthly contribution)
  - Linda's (Mom) IRA value: 82,000 ($500/monthly contribution)
  - Checking/Savings: $12,000
  - Business value: $120,000
  - Vehicles (2) value: $32,000

- **Debt:**
  - Home mortgage: $80,000 ($380/monthly payment)
  - Vehicle debt: $15,000 ($225/monthly payment)
  - Installment debt: $3,600 ($200/monthly payment)
  - Credit card debt: $4,000 ($300/monthly payment)
  - Federal income taxes paid is approximately $31,825 annually or $2,652 monthly
  - Living expenses are approximately $3,000 per month
  - Current college costs are $6,000 per month

Family Goals

- Pay for the cost of undergraduate education as well as mother's NA degree using tax savings and loans.

■ Create enough cash flow by reducing income taxes to make the loan payments on the loans taken out to pay for graduate school.

Tables 5.9 and 5.10 show the family's initial financial situation taken from the preceding financial information and their projected financial situation after implementing some financial strategies.

Columns A and B contain the family's initial financial situation.

■ The initial net cash flow for the family of negative $1,740 is at the bottom of Column B.

The net cash flow is calculated by subtracting "Total Expenses" ($12,552), "Total Asset Contributions" ($1,000), and "Total Liabilities Payments" ($1,105) from "Total Income" ($12,917).

Columns C and D contain the adjustments to the initial financial situation.

1. Linda's income was reduced by $6,667.

2. Because of the income reduction strategies implemented by the parents, their health insurance premiums will be reduced by $400/month.

3. Because of the income reduction strategies implemented by the parents, their children's college costs will decrease by $1,200/month.

4. Because of the income reduction strategies implemented by the parents, their income taxes will decrease by $1,450/month.

5. Discontinue net retirement contributions of $1,000/month.

TABLE 5.9 Family's Initial Financial Situation

	A		B	
	INITIAL ASSET/ LIABILITY		INITIAL MONTHLY CONT/PAYMENT	
Income				
W-2 (Gross)			$	6,667
Interest/Dividends			$	–
Business			$	6,250
Rent			$	–
Other			$	–
Total Income	$	–	$	**12,917**
Expenses				
Health Insurance			$	900
Living Expenses			$	3,000
College			$	6,000
Income Taxes			$	2,652
Total Expenses	$	–	$	**12,552**
Assets				
Retirement	$	137,000	$	1,000
Business	$	120,000	$	–
Residence	$	300,000	$	–
Vehicles	$	32,000	$	–
Other	$	12,000	$	–
Total Assets	$	**601,000**	$	**1,000**
Liabilities				
Home Mortgage	$	80,000	$	380
Vehicle	$	15,000	$	225
Installment	$	3,600	$	200
Credit Card	$	4,000	$	300
Other	$	–	$	–
Total Liabilities	$	**102,600**	$	**1,105**
Net Assets & Cash Flow	$	**486,400**	$	**(1,740)**

TABLE 5.10 Family's Projected Financial Situation

A	B INITIAL ASSET/LIABILITY	C INITIAL MONTHLY CONT/PAYMENT	D MONTHLY CONT/PAYMENT ADJUSTMENT	E ASSET/LIABILITY ADJUSTMENT	F REVISED ASSET/LIABILITY	F REVISED MONTHLY CONT/PAYMENT
Income						
W-2 (Gross)		$ 6,667	$ 6,667			$ 6,667
Interest/Dividends		$ –				$ –
Business		$ 6,250	$ –			$ 6,250
Rent		$ –	$ –			$ –
Other		$ –	$ –			$ –
Total Income	$ –	$ 12,917	$ (6,667)	$ –	$ –	$ 12,917
Expenses						
Health Insurance		$ 900	$ (1) (400)			$ 500
Living Expenses		$ 3,000	$ –			$ 3,000
College		$ 6,000	$ (2) (6,000)			$ 5,100
Income Taxes		$ 2,652	$ (3) (1,650)			$ 1,002
Total Expenses	$ –	$ 12,552	$ (8,050)	$ –	$ –	$ 9,602

Assets							
Retirement	$ 137,000	$ 1,000	$ (1,000)	$ —	$ —	$ —	$ —
Investments	$ —	$ —	$ —	$ —	$ —	$ —	$ —
Business	$ 120,000	$ —	$ —	$ —	$ —	$ —	$ —
Residence	$ 300,000	$ —	$ —	$ —	$ —	$ —	$ —
Vehicles	$ 32,000	$ —	$ —	$ —	$ —	$ —	$ —
Other	$ —	$ —	$ —	$ —	$ —	$ —	$ —
Total Assets	**$ 589,000**	**$ 1,000**	**$ (1,000)**	**$ —**	**$ —**	**$ —**	**$ —**
Liabilities							
Home Mortgage	$ 80,000	$ 380	$ —	$ —	$ —	$ —	$ 380
Vehicle	$ 15,000	$ 225	$ —	$ —	$ —	$ —	$ 225
Installment	$ 3,600	$ 200	$ —	$ —	$ —	$ —	$ 200
Credit Card	$ 4,000	$ 300	$ —	$ —	$ —	$ —	$ 300
Other	$ —	$ —	$ —	$ —	$ —	$ —	$ —
Total Liabilities	**$ 102,600**	**$ 1,105**	**$ —**	**$ —**	**$ —**	**$ —**	**$ 1,105**
Net Assets & Cash Flow	**$ 486,400**	**$ (1,740)**	**$ 2,383**	**$ —**	**$ —**	**$ —**	**$ 643**

Columns E and F contain the revised financial situation.

- The revised net cash flow for the family of $643 is at the bottom of Column F.

- The revised net cash flow is calculated by subtracting "Revised Total Expenses" ($4,562), "Total Revised Asset Contributions" ($0), and "Total Revised Liabilities Payments" ($1,105) from "Total Revised Income" ($6,250).

Bottom Line

Owing to the decrease in health insurance costs, college costs, and income taxes, the family will be able to pay for K-to-12 school costs, undergraduate costs, and incur deferred loans for graduate school. Linda will have to borrow for her degree using Grad PLUS Loans with deferred repayment until after graduation.

CASE STUDY #6

RECENT NURSE PRACTITIONER GRADUATE IN STUDENT LOAN REPAYMENT WHILE SAVING FOR FUTURE HOME PURCHASE

Kathleen is a single 28-year-old recent graduate with her nurse practitioner degree. She has $140,000 in student loan debt and is currently renting an apartment located near her new office at a physicians' group, where her starting salary is $96,000. Kathleen would eventually like to purchase a home, but because of her "millennial mortgage" (a/k/a student loans), she cannot qualify for a home mortgage at this point. She needs to develop a financial plan to help her pay down her student loan debt while saving for a home, retirement, travel, and a new future lifestyle.

Her personal goals are:

1. To pay off her student loan as fast as possible to purchase a house.

2. Create enough cash flow to establish financial security and a better lifestyle.

- **Assets:**
  - 401(k) value: $12,000 ($500/month contribution)
  - Checking/Savings value: $4,000
  - Vehicle value: $34,000
- **Debt:**
  - Vehicle debt: $30,000 ($425/month payment)

- Undergraduate school debt: $40,000 ($265/month payment)

- Graduate school debt: $100,000 ($675/month payment)

- Federal income taxes paid are $1,750/month.

- Health insurance premiums withheld from her paycheck are $200/month

- Living expenses are approximately $4,000/month

Tables 5.11 and 5.12 show her initial financial situation taken from the preceding financial information and her projected financial situation after implementing some financial strategies.

Columns A and B contain her initial financial situation.

- The initial net cash flow is $185 as shown at the bottom of Column B.

- The net cash flow is calculated by subtracting "Total Expenses" ($5,950), "Total Asset Contributions" ($500), and "Total Liabilities Payments" ($1,365) from "Total Income" ($8,000).

TABLE 5.11 Initial Financial Situation

	A		B	
	INITIAL ASSET/ LIABILITY		**INITIAL MONTHLY CONT/PAYMENT**	
Income				
W-2 (Gross)			$	8,000
Interest/Dividends				
Business				
Rent				
Other				
Total Income	$	–	$	**8,000**
Expenses				
Health Insurance			$	200
Living Expenses			$	4,000
College				–
Income Taxes			$	1,750
Total Expenses	$	–	$	**5,950**
Assets				
Retirement	$	12,000	$	500
Residence				
Vehicles	$	34,000		
Other	$	4,000		
Total Assets	$	**50,000**	$	**500**
Liabilities				
Home Mortgage				
Vehicle	$	30,000	$	425
Undergraduate Loan	$	40,000	$	265
Graduate Loan	$	100,000	$	675
Other				
Total Liabilities	$	**170,000**	$	**1,365**
Net Assets/Cash Flow	$	**120,000**	$	**185**

TABLE 5.12 Projected Financial Situation

	A	B	C	D	E	F
	INITIAL ASSET/ LIABILITY	INITIAL MONTHLY CONT/PAYMENT	MONTHLY CONT/PAYMENT ADJUSTMENT	ASSET/ LIABILITY ADJUSTMENT	REVISED ASSET/ LIABILITY	REVISED MONTHLY CONT/PAYMENT
Income						
W-2 (Gross)		$ 8,000	$ –			$ 8,000
Interest/ Dividends						$ –
Business		$ –	$ –			$ –
Rent						$ –
Other		$ –	$ –			$ –
Total Income	$ –	$ 8,000	$ –	$ –	$ –	$ 8,000
Expenses Health Insurance		$ 200	$ –			$ 200
Living Expenses		$ 4,000	$ (1) (250)			$ 3,750
College		$ –	$ –			$ –
Income Taxes		$ 1,750	$ (2) (245)			$ 1,505
Total Expenses	$ –	$ 5,950	$ (495)	$ –	$ –	$ 5,455

Assets						
Retirement	$ 12,000	$ 500	$ –	$ –	$ 12,000	$ 500
Residence	$ –	$ –	$ –	$ –	$ –	$ –
Vehicles	$ 34,000	$ –	$ –	$ –	$ 34,000	$ –
Other	$ 4,000	$ –	$ –	$ –	$ 4,000	$ –
Total Assets	**$ 50,000**	**$ 500**	**$ –**	**$ –**	**$ 50,000**	**$ 500**
Liabilities						
Home Mortgage	$ –	$ –	$ –	$ –	$ –	$ –
Vehicle	$ 30,000	$ 425	$ –	$ –	$ 30,000	$ 425
Installment	$ –	$ –	$ –	$ –	$ –	$ –
Undergraduate Loans	$ 40,000	$ 265	$ –	$ –	$ 40,000	$ 265
Graduate Loans	$ 100,000	$ 675	$ –	$ –	$ 100,000	$ 675
Total Liabilities	**$ 170,000**	**$ 1,365**	**$ –**	**$ –**	**$ 170,000**	**$ 1,365**
Net Assets & Liabilities	**$ (120,000)**	**$ 185**	**$ 495**	**$ –**	**$ (120,000)**	**$ 680**

Columns C and D contain the adjustments to the initial financial situation.

1. As she will receive a $2,500 tax deduction for the student loan interest she is paying, her taxes will be reduced by $45 per month. In addition, her taxes will be reduced by an additional $200 per month because of the home-based business that she started. Therefore, her taxes will be reduced by a total of $245 per month.

2. Living expenses will be reduced by $250 per month after a review of her automobile, renters, professional liability, and disability insurance policies by an independent insurance agent.

Columns E and F contain the revised financial situation.

- The revised net cash flow of $680 per month is at the bottom of Column F.

- The revised net cash flow is calculated by subtracting "Revised Total Expenses" ($5,455), "Total Revised Asset Contributions" ($0), and "Total Revised Liabilities Payments" ($0) from "Total Revised Income" ($8,000).

Financial Strategy

1. Get out of debt
2. Purchase a home (or add to retirement)

Because of her desire to get out of debt and eventually purchase a house (or add to her retirement account), she made $500 per month additional payments on her student loans without changing her current lifestyle.

This allowed her to pay off her student debt in 12 years versus 30 years. At that point in her life, she could use the $940/month that she was previously paying on student loans to make payments on a house, or she could use the money to make additional contributions to her retirement account.

Tables 5.13 and 5.14 illustrate the initial and projected financial situation.

The "Loan Information" section contains the following information:

1. The total student "Loan Amount": $140,000

2. The "Annual Interest Rate": 7.08%

3. The "Number of Monthly Payments": 360 monthly payments

4. The "Monthly Payment Amount": $939/month

The "Extra Payments" section is not used for the initial financial information.

The "Loan Summary" section contains the following information:

1. The "Total of All Payments": $338,025

2. The "Total Interest Paid": $198,025

3. The "Years Until Paid Off": 30 years

4. The "Interest Savings": $0

The "Investment Summary" section in Table 5.14 contains the following information:

1. The "Current Age": 28 years old

TABLE 5.13 Initial Financial Situation

Loan Information	
Loan Amount	$140,000
Annual Interest Rate	7.080%
Number of Monthly Payments	360
Monthly Payment Amount	**$938.96**
Extra Payments	
Extra Monthly Payment	
Extra Annual Payment	
Month of Annual Payment	
Total Extra Payments	**$0.00**
Loan Summary	
Total of All Payments	$338,024.69
Total Interest Paid	$198,024.69
Years Until Paid Off	30.00
Interest Savings	**$0.00**

TABLE 5.14 Projected Financial Situation

INVESTMENT SUMMARY	
Current Age	28
Retirement Age	68
Investment per Year	
Rate of Return	5.00%
Years Until Paid in Full	30.00
Value of Investment @ Paid in Full	**$0.00**
Number of Years Until Retirement	10.00
Extra Payment per Year	
Monthly Loan Payment	$938.96
Balance at Retirement	**$145,803.46**

2. The "Retirement Age": 68 years old

3. The "Rate of Return": 5% return on retirement assets

4. The "Years Until Paid in Full": 30 years

5. The "Number of Years Until Retirement": 10 years

6. The "Monthly Loan Payment": $939/month put into retirement account

7. The "Balance at Retirement": $145,803 addition to retirement account

The "Loan Information" section in Table 5.15 contains the following information:

1. The total student "Loan Amount": $140,000

2. The "Annual Interest Rate": 7.08%

3. The "Number of Monthly Payments": 360 monthly payments

4. The "Monthly Payment Amount": $939/month

The "Extra Payments" section contains the following information:

1. The "Extra Monthly Payments": $500/month on the student loans

2. The "Total Extra Payments": $72,500 over a 12-year period

The "Loan Summary" section contains the following information:

5. The "Total of All Payments": $208,745

6. The "Total Interest Paid": $68,745

7. The "Years Until Paid Off": 12.17 years

8. The "Interest Savings": $129,280

The "Investment Summary" section contains the following information:

9. The "Current Age": 28 years old

10. The "Retirement Age": 68 years old

11. The "Rate of Return": 5% return on retirement assets

12. The "Years Until Paid in Full": 12.17 years

13. The "Number of Years Until Retirement": 27.83 years to retirement after the loans are paid off

14. The "Monthly Loan Payment: $939/month put into retirement account

15. The "Balance at Retirement": $692,721 addition to retirement account

Bottom Line

When the student loans are paid off in 12 years, she will then have the option to buy a house or put her money into a retirement account and have an additional $692,720 in her retirement account when she retires (Tables 5.15 and 5.16).

TABLE 5.15 Extra Payments and Loan Summary

Loan Information	
Loan Amount	$140,000
Annual Interest Rate	7.080%
Number of Monthly Payments	360
Monthly Payment Amount	**$938.96**
Extra Payments	
Extra Monthly Payment	$500
Extra Annual Payment	
Month of Annual Payment	
Total Extra Payments	**$72,500.00**
Loan Summary	
Total of All Payments	$208,745.09
Total Interest Paid	$68,745.09
Years Until Paid Off	12.17
Interest Savings	**$129,279.60**

TABLE 5.16 Investment Summary for Retirement

INVESTMENT SUMMARY	
Current Age	28
Retirement Age	68
Investment per Year	
Rate of Return	5.00%
Years Until Paid in Full	12.17
Value of Investment @ Paid in Full	**$0.00**
Number of Years Until Retirement	27.83
Extra Payment per Year	
Monthly Loan Payment	$938.96
Balance at Retirement	**$692,720.77**

APPENDIX

CHECKLIST FOR COLLEGE FUNDING OPPORTUNITIES

1. Only use your tax return information from the prior-prior year (PPY), not the prior year, when submitting your FAFSA.

2. Does your grad school also require your parent's information for financial aid analysis? Believe it or not, some do.

3. Is your grad school financial aid offer satisfactory? If not, consider appealing for a better offer (in-person, if possible).

4. Compare and contrast both federal and private loans for the best "deal," especially with regard to interest rates and flexible repayment plans.

5. Always ask about grad school institutional scholarships, meaning from the colleges you have applied to.

6. How, when, and why to appeal is covered in the book; use the tips for your unique needs.

7. When applying for financial aid, ask whether there are any (additional) forms you need to complete besides the FAFSA.

8. Always ask the grad school financial aid office what the full cost of attendance per year is, and whether your financial aid award is expected to remain the same from year to year.

9. Ask the grad school aid counselor: On average, how much do nursing students borrow from their institution to earn their grad nursing degree?

10. If possible, speak to other nursing grad students at the college you are applying to for their "inside" tips.

TOP 10 NURSING SCHOLARSHIP RESOURCES

1. The Emergency Nursing Association (ENA) offers annual academic scholarships up to doctoral degrees: https://www.ena.org/foundation/scholarships

2. The American Cancer Association offers graduate scholarships for students pursuing an MSN or Doctorate of Nursing Practice (DNP) specializing in oncology: https://www.cancer.org/research/we-fund-cancer-research/apply-research-grant/grant-types/graduate-scholarships-cancer-nursing.html

3. The Nurses Education Funds offer several scholarships to nurses pursuing advanced nursing degrees: https://www.n-e-f.org/about/nef-scholarships.html

4. The Health Resources and Services Administration funds nursing education programs: https://bhw.hrsa.gov/grants/nursing

5. Johnson & Johnson offers nursing funding opportunities and scholarship search: https://nursing.jnj.com/scholarships?f0=00000165-9052-d24d-a3fd-d652ec1d0000

6. The American Association of Nurse Practitioners (AANP) provides financial support to nursing students to advance their NP education: https://www.nursepractitionerschools.com/blog/np-scholarships

7. Graduate nursing students can find financial aid and scholarship and repayment information at: www.collegescholarships.org/graduate-nursing.htm

8. Continuing professional development scholarships are available through the American Association of Critical Care Nurses: https://www.aacn.org/education/scholarship

9. The March of Dimes offers scholarships to graduate nursing students enrolled in programs of maternal–child nursing: https://www.marchofdimes.org/professionals/graduate-nursing-scholarships.aspx

10. The Nurse Practitioner Healthcare Foundation (NPHF) offers award to nurse practitioners in the field of gastroenterology: https://www.nphealthcarefoundation.org/scholarships-awards-fellowships/gastroenterology

FINANCIAL RESOURCES
FOR NURSING STUDENTS

https://nursejournal.org/articles/nursing-scholarships
-grants

- **NURSE Corps:** The NURSE Corps offers loan repayment programs and scholarship opportunities in exchange for service in underserved communities. Recipients must commit to working for at least two years in underserved areas or facilities with critical staffing needs.

- **New Graduate Residency Programs:** This database from the Columbia University School of Nursing includes information on nursing residency and fellowship programs across the country.

- **Health Resources and Services Administration:** This administration provides information on federal and state loan repayment and forgiveness programs. Students can also use it to learn more about underserved areas through the comprehensive fact sheets and data collections.

- **American Nurses Foundation:** The American Nurses Foundation provides funding for research grants, fellowships, scholarships, and more. Much of the organization's scholarship funding filters down to state associations, allowing donors to support nurses across the country.

- **Federal Student Aid:** Learn about completing the FAFSA, as well as grant programs and loan opportunities available through the U.S. Department of Education. The site also offers information on choosing a school and avoiding scholarship and loan scams.

INVESTMENTS FOR DEFERRING INCOME TO COLLEGE YEARS

There are several investments to defer income to college years to take advantage of a child's tax capacity. One or a combination of the following investments may be used to defer income to college years.

1. Coverdell Education Savings Accounts
2. Qualified tuition plans
3. I bonds and EE bonds
4. Traditional IRAs and SIMPLE IRAs
5. Roth IRAs
6. Tax-efficient funds
7. Annuities
8. Life insurance
9. Real estate

ASSET STRATEGIES FOR FINANCIAL AID-ELIGIBLE FAMILIES WITH A CHILD IN COLLEGE

1. The family should inquire about the college's policy concerning annuities and the cash value of life insurance before considering the

purchase of these investments. Some private colleges, usually the most elite ones, assess these assets.

2. If the child earns, he may consider saving for college by purchasing a Roth IRA.

3. As retirement accounts are not assessed in the expected family contribution (EFC) formulas, saving for college using retirement accounts and then borrowing against the accounts to pay for college may be a viable strategy.

4. If the family plans a purchase in the near future, it may be wise to use an assessable asset, such as cash, to purchase a nonassessable personal asset, such as a personal computer.

5. Personal debt cannot be used to reduce the net worth of an assessable asset. However, personal items, such as cars, boats, motorcycles, or jewelry, are not considered as assets in the financial aid formula.

6. The family should consider paying down personal debt with an assessable asset (savings).

7. Claiming a second home interest expense deduction on Schedule A for a boat or motor home makes these assessable assets.

8. As the Federal Methodology (FM) formula does not assess family farm assets, the family may consider using nonfarm assessable assets, such as certificates of deposit (CDs), to pay down farm-related debt.

9. The family may want to delay signing the financial aid applications until after the older

parent's birthday. Under the FM formula, this will increase the "Asset Protection Allowance."

10. If the family has assets subject to a life estate, the family should appeal to the Financial Aid Administrator (FAA), because these assets cannot be liquidated to pay for college costs.

11. If the family has assets tied up in probate, the family should appeal to the FAA if there will be no distribution of assets during college years.

12. The family can reduce the value of a trust by spending the trust assets for the benefit of the student (e.g., trust buys a car for college or pays for the student's private high school tuition). If the family takes assets out of a trust or custodial account and the assets are not used for the benefit of the student, there can be some adverse legal and tax consequences.

13. If the family's child's access to trust funds is restricted until after college years, the value of the trust should be appealed to the FAA.

14. If the family's child is the beneficiary of a Qualified Tuition Plan (QTP) and qualifies for financial aid, the family should consider rolling the QTP to another beneficiary.

15. If the family qualifies for the "Simplified EFC" exception, neither the family's assets nor those of the student will be assessed in the FM formula.

16. If the family qualifies for the "Zero EFC" exception, the student will automatically have a zero EFC.

17. The Institutional Methodology formula will also assess the student's siblings' assets, at the parents' assessment rate.

18. On what date would the value of the assets be the least? If possible, the financial aid application form should be signed on the date the assets are at their least value.

ASSET STRATEGIES FOR UPPER-INCOME FAMILIES

1. Funding a life insurance policy over a period of several years could be a viable option. It can allow the family to take maximum advantage of tax-deferred growth and tax-advantaged withdrawals for college, as well as retirement.

2. Gifts that families pay directly to an educational institution (either elementary and high school or college) for their child's tuition will not reduce the annual $14,000 gift tax exclusion for that child. The gifts must be made directly to the educational institution.

3. If families wanted to transfer more funds to their child or grandchild than the annual $14,000 gift exclusion, they could accomplish this by making a loan to the child for the amount in excess of the $14,000 gift exclusion limit. They would then forgive up to $14,000 per year until the loan balance is zero.

4. There is a special rule for contributions to a QTP that exceed the annual gift tax exclusion.

If a contribution in excess of the annual $14,000 gift tax exclusion is made in one year, the family may elect to have the contribution treated as if made ratably over five years.

5. Charitable remainder trusts can produce a double tax saving, which can be used to help fund college costs. In a typical charitable remainder trust, you would donate a remainder interest in an asset to a charity. The family would receive a current charitable donation tax deduction, remove the asset from their estate, and retain an income interest in the asset to help fund college costs.

6. A highly appreciated low-yielding asset can be contributed to a charitable remainder trust.

7. As the charitable remainder trust is exempt from taxation, the asset can be sold tax-free. The proceeds can then be reinvested in a higher-yielding investment without depleting the investment principal.

8. The Roth IRA is an attractive vehicle to use for college, with benefits such as the tax and penalty-free withdrawal of original contributions.

9. A grandparent can will his Roth IRA to his grandchild. The minimum distribution rules will require distributions from the Roth IRA to be based on the life expectancy of the grandchild. The grandchild could take minimum distributions (the balance of the account continues to grow tax-free) until college years and then withdraw additional tax-free funds for college.

10. A Voluntary Employees' Beneficiary Association (VEBA) can allow for large, flexible, and fully tax-deductible contributions. The assets accumulate and compound on a tax-deferred basis while remaining protected from both personal and corporate creditors.

11. If additional funds for college are needed, you should consider a federal Parent's Loan for Undergraduate Students (PLUS loan). A PLUS loan is a signature loan with an interest rate capped at 9%. These loans can be made only for undergraduate college expenses.

12. If additional funds for college are needed, the family should consider having their child obtain an unsubsidized Stafford loan. As an unsubsidized Stafford loan is in the child's name, the child can deduct the student loan interest expense. Also, if the family cannot deduct student loan interest expense (because of the income limitations), an unsubsidized Stafford loan in the student's name is preferable to a PLUS loan in the family's name.

13. If additional funds for college are needed, the family should consider having their child obtain an alternative student loan in the student's name. If the loan is in the student's name, the student can deduct the student loan interest expense. Because of the deductible interest expense, these loans may be preferable to a PLUS loan in the family's name.

14. The family can either use an equity line of credit or a second mortgage on a residence for

college funds. The interest paid can be deducted as an itemized deduction.

15. The family can borrow, up to a certain amount, from their retirement account, if the account allows borrowing. Usually, the interest rate and repayment terms are favorable. However, if the family member with this account loses this job, the outstanding loan balance may have to be immediately repaid, or taxable income will occur. Also, if the loans are not repaid within a certain time period, usually five years, the outstanding principal balance becomes taxable.

16. The family could loan money to their child for college. The family would receive payments on the loan from their child. The difference between the rate of return the family is receiving on the money loaned to their child and the interest rate their child would have paid from an outside source could be used to reduce the family's cost of college.

17. The deduction for alimony creates an opportunity to shift income from a higher to a lower tax bracket spouse. Additional payments that can be considered alimony are medical insurance and other expenditures, such as mortgage payments, real estate taxes, insurance, utilities, life insurance premiums, and college expenses, made on behalf of a former spouse under a divorce decree or separation agreement.

18. Under the financial aid rules for divorce or separation situations, the income and assets of only the custodial parent are used to compute

a child's eligibility for financial aid. (Note: Some private colleges also factor in the income and assets of the noncustodial parent.) Therefore, the family should carefully consider with whom the child will live during college years.

19. The family can use a 401(k) wraparound plan to put excess 401(k) contributions into a nonqualified plan. These excess contributions can be used to fund a child's future college costs. The family does not have to report taxable income before the excess contributions are put into the nonqualified plan. The family must make two separate elections: (1) to contribute to the 401(k) plan, and (2) to have the excess contributions transferred to the nonqualified plan.

INCOME STRATEGIES FOR FINANCIAL AID-ELIGIBLE FAMILIES

1. As loan proceeds are not assessed, it may be better to borrow funds during college years rather than attempting to pay for college by striving to increase earnings, which decreases financial aid eligibility.

2. The student should avoid cash gifts from people other than parents during college years, as these are treated as "untaxed income" in the financial aid system. If cash gifts are going to be given to the student, they should be given in noncollege years. Alternatively, loans could be given to the student during college years,

and then a cash gift could be given to repay the loan after college years.

3. Cash gifts, which are paid directly to the college for tuition and fees (from people other than the parents), should be avoided. These gifts are treated as a student "resource" and create a dollar-for-dollar deduction in financial aid.

4. As the current year's contribution to a retirement plan is assessed as "untaxed income," the family should maximize contributions to a retirement plan during noncollege years and minimize contributions during college years.

5. Parents should avoid withdrawals from retirement, pension, annuity, or life insurance plans during college years because both the interest, included in the Adjusted Gross Income (AGI), and the principal withdrawal, included as "untaxed income," will be assessed. If withdrawals of assessable assets are made, an assessment of this withdrawal should be appealed to the FAA. The appeal should be based on the fact that the transfer of principal from one type of asset to another type of asset does not create an additional source of funds to pay for college.

6. If a taxable conversion from a Regular IRA to a Roth IRA is made, the assessment of this taxable rollover income should be appealed to the FAA. Remember that nontaxable rollovers are not assessed.

7. Eligibility for the Employment Expense Allowance deduction is allowed only if both parents have earned income. Therefore, both

spouses should have earned income to qualify for this allowance; this could be accomplished by hiring a nonworking spouse in the family business.

8. The family should consider having the family's business establish a medical reimbursement plan (IRC Sec. 105) for an employee-spouse to shift medical expenses from Schedule A to the business schedule, and consequently, lower the family's AGI.

9. The student's income should be kept at approximately $6,000 during college years. Shifting income to the student should be considered if the student does not have this much income. This will lower the parents' AGI without having a negative effect on the student's financial aid eligibility.

10. Wages from closely held entities should be kept down during college years.

11. Minimize the amount of state or local tax refunds during college years. To ensure that refunds are not received, accurate withholding or estimated payments should be made.

12. Consider accelerating or postponing capital asset purchases during college years to lower business income through depreciation or additional first year depreciation (AFYD) on the capital asset.

13. The family should consider accelerating tax-deductible expenses during college years.

14. The family should consider obtaining commercial bank loans rather than taxable Commodity Credit Corporation (CCC) loans (farmers) during college years.

15. The family should consider selling stocks in noncollege years that would generate capital gain distributions during college years.

16. Avoid income distributions from estates or trusts during college years.

17. The family should consider not itemizing tax deductions during college years.

INCOME STRATEGIES FOR UPPER-INCOME FAMILIES

1. Outright gifts of appreciated assets to the child or grandchild may be an effective way to shift income and assets to the child or grandchild. Significant income and estate tax savings can be achieved by outright gifts. However, control of assets that are gifted outright to the child or grandchild will be lost immediately.

2. When a family's income reaches a certain level, all or part of their personal exemptions is phased out. Therefore, they would not receive any tax benefit from their child's personal exemption. However, if the child can show that he, and not the family, is providing over half of his support, he can claim the personal exemption on his tax return.

3. If the family is at least in the 25% tax bracket, they should consider gifting appreciated assets to their child (over age 24) and then have the child sell the asset. If the child is in the 15% tax bracket, his capital gains rate would be a 0% rate, as opposed to the family's 15% capital gains rate.

4. Families can receive tax benefits if they employ their child. As the child receives "earned" income, he is not subject to the "kiddie tax," even if he is less than 24 years of age. Also, because it is earned income, the child will be able to utilize his standard deduction. Another benefit of a child having earned income is that he can contribute to a Roth or regular IRA for future college costs.

5. A family member can hire his or her spouse in their business and establish a medical reimbursement plan for the spouse and the rest of their family. In effect, this would turn non-deductible medical expenses into deductible business expenses.

6. A family limited partnership can provide the family with a way to shift income to their children and reduce their estate. Typically, in a family limited partnership, the family is the general partner and their children the limited partners. The limited partners cannot make investment, business, or management decisions. The family would make annual gifts of partnership interests to their children.

7. A sale or gift to and subsequent leaseback from a child can be used to shift income to the

child, but be aware of the kiddie tax rules. The family could sell or gift property to their child with a simultaneous leaseback from the child. The sale or gift may be made directly to the child or in trust for the child.

8. A family may gift the maximum amount allowed by the annual gift tax exclusion ($13,000) and take a note from their child for the balance of the funds needed for college. Then, instead of the child having to make payments on the note, the parent could forgive a portion of the principal (and interest) each year equal to the annual gift tax exclusion.

9. A QTP can be used to shift income to a child or grandchild. The income generated from assets gifted to a QTP grows tax-deferred. When the child receives distributions from the QTP for college, the accumulated income is tax-free to him.

10. Tax shelters are a form of deferring income. One of the best tax shelters for college is an oil and gas investment. As a general rule, the tax write-off on an oil and gas investment does not exceed 100% of the amount of the investment. Working interests in oil and gas ventures are generally not treated as passive activities.

11. As the kiddie tax applies to unearned income of a child under 24 years of age, one strategy to avoid the kiddie tax is to invest the child's assets in investments, such as municipal bonds

or growth stocks, which generate tax-exempt or tax-deferred income until the child reaches age 24.

12. A parent can elect to have the interest on their child's U.S. EE savings bonds taxed each year and, if the child is not subject to the kiddie tax, the interest will be taxed at his lower tax rates. Therefore, in the year that a child redeems the bonds, he will not have to pay any tax on the proceeds.

13. A family's business can establish a fringe benefit program for their child/employee. If the type of fringe benefit established by the business is tax-deductible and taxable to a child/employee (e.g., employer-provided automobile), this causes an income-shifting effect. If the type of fringe benefit established by the business is deductible by a business but not taxable to a child/employee (e.g., medical reimbursement), the tax savings can be used to cut the cost of college.

HOUSEHOLD STRATEGIES FOR FINANCIAL AID FAMILIES

1. The financial aid application should be signed on the date when the household status is the most beneficial.

2. If the student's parents are divorced, the income and assets of the parent with whom the student lived the most in the last 12 months

must be reported. Therefore, the income and assets of the parent with whom the student lives with during college years must be considered.

3. If the student's parents are divorced and the student lived equally with the parents (e.g., joint custody), the income and assets of the parent who provided the most support in the last 12 months must be reported. Therefore, the income and assets of the parent who provides the most support during college years must be considered.

4. When structuring a divorce agreement, it may be better to give the custodial parent more assets and less income.

5. If the student has a stepparent, the income and assets of the stepparent must be reported. Therefore, the timing of the signing of the financial aid application and the marriage of the parent/stepparent should be considered.

6. To list a child who is not living with the parent as a member of the household, the parent should provide more than half the support of that child.

7. If the child does not meet one of the criteria to be automatically considered an "independent student" but is financially independent of the parent and does not live with the parent, the student can appeal to the FAA for "independent student" status.

EDUCATION TAX INCENTIVE STRATEGIES FOR ALL FAMILIES

1. If the parents' AGI is too high to claim the American Opportunity Credit (AOC) or Lifetime Learning Credit (LLC), the parents should consider giving up the exemption for the student so that the student can claim the AOC or LC. The student cannot claim the exemption unless he is providing more than half of his support.

2. The timing of the payment of qualified expenses may ensure that the maximum AOC or LLC can be claimed.

3. If a college does not have a set payment ordering system for tax-free grants and scholarships, the parent can arrange for the payments of nontuition and fee expenses to be eligible for the AOC or LC. (This causes all or a portion of the scholarship to be taxable.)

4. Withdrawals from an IRA during years in which the student is eligible for financial aid should be avoided.

5. A family with two students in college at the same time could consider giving up the exemption for one of the students, so that one student can claim the LLC and the parents could claim the LLC for the other student. Therefore, the family could claim two LLCs.

6. The AOC or LLC can be claimed by the taxpayer who claims the student as a dependent, even if the college expenses are actually paid by the student or by a third party.

7. Parents whose AGI is too high to make a contribution to a Coverdell Education Savings Account (CESA) can make a gift to other persons, who can then make the contribution.

8. The student should consider delaying the withdrawal of CESA funds until after December 31 of the final year of college. CESA accounts are assessed as an asset of the parents in the financial aid formulas.

9. Qualified tuition plans (QTPs) can be an effective method of shifting income to a child on a tax-free basis.

10. QTPs can be used as a vehicle to defer income

11. In certain states QTPs may be exempt from state taxation.

12. In certain states, QTP contributions may be deductible for state income tax purposes.

13. QTPs can be used to reduce estates without giving up control of the asset. The owner of the account can withdraw the account funds, subject to income taxes and penalty. A five-year averaging of the gift is allowed.

14. QTP accounts can be rolled over to another beneficiary if the current beneficiary is eligible for financial aid.

15. The parents need to consider the financial aid impact of QTPs when deciding whether to purchase them and what type to purchase (i.e., prepaid vs. college savings).

16. Interest paid on loans from relatives does not qualify for the student loan interest deduction.

17. Student loan interest cannot be deducted until the interest is repaid.

18. If the parents' AGI is too high to claim a student loan interest deduction, the student could take a Federal Unsubsidized Stafford loan or a private loan in the student's name and deduct the interest.

19. The timing of repayment of student loans to increase the student loan interest deduction should be considered.

20. Parents who are ineligible for the student loan interest deduction may consider taking out a deductible home mortgage loan.

21. If withdrawals from regular or Roth IRAs are needed to pay for college, the withdrawal should be timed to occur during college years to escape the 10% early withdrawal penalty.

APPEAL STRATEGIES FOR ALL FAMILIES

1. If a college's financial aid award offer does not meet a family's expectations, either in the amount of the offer or in the type of aid offered (gift-aid vs. self-help aid), the family should appeal to the FAA. Do not ask to "negotiate" with the FAA; the word "negotiate" offends some FAAs. Ask to "appeal" an award offer.

2. The FAA has the authority to change the information reported on the financial aid applications in any way that the FAA thinks will

more clearly reflect a family's ability to pay for college. This authority is called "professional judgment."

3. The family must have specific reasons why they need more financial aid. These reasons are known as "special circumstances." The special circumstances should be adequately documented to make it easy for the FAA to say "yes" to the appeal.

4. Special circumstances may include:

   - Death
   - Divorce/separation
   - Disability or injury
   - Unemployment
   - Sickness, medical, or handicap expense
   - Natural disasters
   - Dislocated worker
   - Unusually high child-care expenses
   - Unreimbursed expenses shown on Form 2106
   - One-time bonus
   - Unusually high income
   - Unusually low expenses

5. An appeal should request a specific amount of increased financial aid.

6. In most cases, an FAA considers an appeal only if a financial aid application or Student Aid Report has been filed or received by the FAA.

INVESTMENT STRATEGIES FOR ALL FAMILIES

1. U.S. Series EE bonds are tax-deferred or tax-free (when used to pay qualified education expenses), low-risk investments that can be used as part of the long-term college financial aid plan.

2. Zero coupon bonds are currently taxed investments that lock in the current rate of interest and a specific amount on maturity. They can be used as part of the long-term college financial plan.

3. Municipal bonds are tax-free, low-risk investments that lock in the interest rate. They can be used as part of the long-term college financial plan.

4. Mutual funds are growth-oriented long-term investments that allow for the switching of investments without incurring sales charges. They can be used as part of the long-term college financial plan.

5. QTPs are tax-deferred, and possibly tax-free, accounts that are used to pay for tuition, fees, and room and board at the colleges specified in the investment contract. The gifts to these accounts can be spread over five years, which allows for large one-time gifts to these programs. As the owner of the account can switch beneficiaries, the owner can maintain some control over the funds.

6. A Roth IRA is a long-term investment that grows tax-deferred. The withdrawals made

from these accounts after age 59½ are tax- and penalty-free. The nondeductible original contributions may be withdrawn tax-free for any use. In addition, there is no 10% early withdrawal penalty on withdrawals made before age 59½ that are used to pay qualified college expenses.

7. Traditional IRAs may be tax-deferred long-term investments. They can be withdrawn penalty-free (10% penalty for withdrawal before age 59½) to pay for qualified college expenses. The contributions to these accounts are tax deductible.

8. Real estate is a long-term growth-oriented investment the appreciation of which grows tax-deferred in value and is taxed at the favorable capital gains rate when sold. If the real estate is rented, it may generate significant tax losses (through depreciation).

OTHER COST-CUTTING STRATEGIES FOR FAMILIES WITH COLLEGE STUDENTS

1. The Internet has several sites that offer discounts to students for books, travel, and so on.

2. The student can participate in a three-year degree program that allows him to complete a bachelor's degree in three years, while pursuing a masters or doctorate.

3. The student can attend a college with a guaranteed four-year degree program (guarantees graduation in four years).

4. Some colleges offer programs that allow the student to attend five years of college for the cost of four years.

5. Some colleges offer programs that combine undergraduate with graduate studies in one degree.

6. Some colleges offer a guaranteed tuition price for four years.

7. Some colleges offer financing programs that help families spread out tuition payments.

8. Some colleges offer tuition reduction plans that are excluded from gross income, if used for undergraduate courses.

9. The student can attend a community or junior college and obtain a college degree without a huge cost.

10. The student can attend a low-cost community (junior) college for one or two years and then shift to a private college and earn a degree from a prestigious private college.

11. The student can reduce costs by taking advanced placement (AP) courses in high school and earn college credit, which reduces the time spent in college.

ALTERNATIVE WAYS TO REDUCE COSTS FOR FAMILIES WITH A COLLEGE-BOUND STUDENT

Let us quickly examine some more innovative payment options in case you did not get enough money for your child's college education. Or, if you are the parent of a high school junior, these payment options will help you understand where to turn if the schools let you down and you still need more money for college.

Some schools, particularly the private universities, have more flexibility when it comes to negotiating for a better financial aid package, whereas others, such as state colleges, have very little room to do anything. This makes it imperative for you, as a parent, to understand all the payment options available to you just in case the college your child has her heart set on offers less than you expect or need when awarding your financial aid.

- **Have Your Child Start Out at a State School and Then Transfer to a Private College**

  - If your child is accepted at both private universities and state schools, and she prefers to go to one of the private schools, the first thing you need to look at is how much it is really going to cost you to send her to that school. If the private university offers you an excellent package, which approximately costs you the same whether you send your child to private or state, simply send your child to her top choice.

  - If, however, the private university offers you a less than competitive package and sending your child there will put you deep into debt, think about sending her to a state school for two years and then have her transfer over to a private university.

- You will probably end up saving yourself about $30,000, and your child will end up with a diploma from a private university. However, it is important to realize that if your child does not get top grades (A– or higher) at the state school, she is going to have a tough time transferring over to a top private university. Also, schools tend not to offer their best packages to transfer students, but it may balance out due to the tuition savings.

- **Think About Sending Your Child to a College That Offers Cooperative Education**

  - About 900 colleges and universities across the country offer programs where students can alternate between full-time study and a full-time job. This differs from work–study in that work–study jobs tend to be jobs that students are not interested in for a couple of hours a day until they have earned the amount of the award.

  - However, cooperative education offers periods of full-time employment in jobs that the student is interested in pursuing after she graduates. The student usually makes enough money to pay for a good portion of tuition and she has a much better chance of landing a good job after graduation. The only downside is it usually takes 5 years to graduate, but it may be well worth it as, in addition to the degree the student holds, she will also have valuable, real-world experience. Tip: Co-op earnings do not count against need-based financial aid eligibility.

- **Have Your Child Take the Military Route**

  - There are two different options. The first one is the Reserve Officer Training Corps (ROTC), which has branches at many colleges. To qualify for an ROTC scholarship, which usually covers full or partial tuition plus $100 a month allowance, your child must apply in her senior year of high school. He or she should also have good grades and 1,200 (verbal and math) or above SAT scores.

  - The other option is applying to one of the service academies, which are extremely difficult to get into. To apply, your child must have excellent grades and SAT scores, pass a physical, and have a recommendation from a congressperson or senator. If your child can fulfill all of the aforementioned requirements, she will enjoy a *free* college education.

  - The only downside of going the military route is that your child will be required to serve several years in the military after graduation.

- **Try Borrowing From an Innovative Loan Program**

  - Before you look into any type of loan programs, do your best to qualify for federally subsidized loans that are interest free and principal free until your child graduates. If you still need to borrow more money, try borrowing from your 401(k) plan or a pension plan. Many plans will allow you to borrow up to 50% of the value of the plan or up to $50,000 interest free. You should also think about taking out a home equity loan instead of a commercial loan, as your interest payments may be tax-deductible.

- Locate and apply for every "need-based" scholarship, grant, and low-interest loan.

- Find, or get help finding, all the "need-based" sources of funding through the federal government, the state you live in, and the colleges and universities your child is applying to (in-state or out-of-state schools). Most of these financial aid programs can be applied for by simply filling out the federal form (the FAFSA) and, in some cases, the Institutional Form (which is the College Board's CSS Profile that is used at about 300 colleges).

- **Send Your Child to a Community College for the First Two Years of School**

  - If your child works hard and gets good grades, she can usually transfer to a top private university. This way, she can get a diploma from a prestigious school for half the cost.

  - Choose colleges that have innovative payment plans.

- Do not only pay attention to the normal college search criteria such as courses offered, academic and athletic reputation, geographic location, and so on. Instead, make sure you inquire about special scholarships, installment plans, guaranteed cost plans, and tuition reductions for good grades.

- **Have Your Child Complete Four Years of College in Three Years**

  - Your child will have to attend summer school, but you will save the 7% to 8% increase in tuition for the fourth year.

- **Have Your Child Enroll in Advanced Placement Classes or Enroll in College-Level Courses While She Is Still in High School**

  - Every college-level course the child takes in high school is one less course to pay for when the child goes to college. Considering college credits can cost as much as $300 each, having your child place out of these courses can save you money.

- **Tuition Reductions**

  - According to a tuition reduction executive summary released by the National Association of College and University Business Officers, the nation's private colleges continue to discount the price of acquiring an education. Many private colleges offer discounts to stay competitive with lower-cost state colleges, because private colleges receive little or no support from state tax dollars.

■ Tuition reductions come from many private colleges' own institutional funds and are given to students in the form of a merit grant and scholarship. In other words, the college discounts its "sticker price" to help attract students to its institution, regardless of the family's income level and qualifications for need-based financial aid.

■ Tuition reductions allow many private colleges to compete with lower-cost public universities for the best students. In many cases, these discounts will lower tuition costs into the same price range as a public university. Families looking for a quality college education at a reduced cost should apply to these lesser-known private schools.

■ It is important for the parents to ask for information on merit grants and scholarships and other incentives at these private colleges, as they differ from college to college.

■ If the student is attending an out-of-state college, establish residency in that state in order to pay in-state tuition. In addition, see if your institution has a reciprocity agreement with other nearby states.

■ Distance learning can be used to earn college credits.

BIBLIOGRAPHY

All Nursing Schools. (n.d.). Top 10 most common questions about online nursing school. Retrieved from https://www.all nursingschools.com/articles/online-nursing-school

American Association of Colleges of Nursing. (2017). *The numbers behind the degree*. Retrieved from http://www.aacnnursing.org/ Portals/42/Policy/PDF/Debt_Report.pdf

American Association of Critical Care Nurses. (n.d.). *AACN continuing professional development scholarships*. Retrieved from https://www.aacn.org/education/scholarship

American Association of Nurse Practitioners. (n.d.). *50 top NP scholarships*. Retrieved from https://www.nursepractitioner schools.com/blog/np-scholarships

American Cancer Society. (n.d.). *Graduate scholarships in cancer nursing practice*. Retrieved from https://www.cancer.org/ research/we-fund-cancer-research/apply-research-grant/grant -types/graduate-scholarships-cancer-nursing.html

American Nurses Foundation. (2019). Retrieved from https://www .nursingworld.org/foundation

Boyington, B., & Moody, J. (2019). Top colleges, universities for internships, co-ops. *U.S. News*. Retrieved from https://www .usnews.com/education/best-colleges/slideshows/top-colleges -universities-for-internship-co-op-programs?onepage

College Scholarship Search. (n.d.). *Find nursing scholarships and nursing education loan repayment*. Retrieved from http://www .collegescholarships.org/graduate-nursing.htm

Columbia University School of Nursing. (2019). *New graduate residency programs*. Retrieved from http://www.nursing.columbia .edu/students/career-development/new-graduate-residency -programs

Credit Union Student Choice. (2019). *Student loan refinancing*. Retrieved from https://www.studentchoice.org/borrow/student -loan-refinance/

Davis, N. P. (2013). *The 2013 NACUBO tuition discounting study*. Washington, DC: National Association of College and

University Business Officers. Retrieved from https://www.iwu
.edu/associate-provost/2013_tds_final_report.pdf

Emergency Nursing Association. (n.d.). *Scholarships.* Retrieved
from https://www.ena.org/foundation/scholarships

Federal Student Aid. (n.d.). *Loan consolidation.* Retrieved from
https://studentaid.ed.gov/sa/repay-loans/consolidation

Federal Student Aid. (n.d.). *Public service loan forgiveness.*
Retrieved from https://studentaid.ed.gov/sa/repay-loans/forgive
ness-cancellation/public-service#qualify

Federal Student Aid. (2019). Retrieved from https://studentaid.ed
.gov/sa

Health Resources & Services Administration. (n.d.). About Nurse
Corps. Retrieved from https://bhw.hrsa.gov/loans-scholarships/
nurse-corps/about-nurse-corps

Health Resources & Services Administration. (n.d.). *Grants:
Nursing.* Retrieved from https://bhw.hrsa.gov/grants/nursing

Health Resources & Services Administration. (n.d.). *School-based
loans and scholarships.* Retrieved from https://bhw.hrsa.gov/
loansscholarships/schoolbasedloans

Internal Revenue Service. (2019). *Tax benefits for education:
Information center.* Retrieved from https://www.irs.gov/
newsroom/tax-benefits-for-education-information-center

Johnson & Johnson. (2019). *Paying for school.* Retrieved from
https://nursing.jnj.com/scholarships

March of Dimes. (n.d.). *Graduate nursing scholarships.* Retrieved from
https://www.marchofdimes.org/professionals/graduate-nursing
-scholarships.aspx

Nurse Journal. (n.d.). *Financial aid overview and scholarships.*
Retrieved from https://nursejournal.org/articles/nursing-scholar
ships-grants

Nurse Practitioner Healthcare Foundation. (2019). *Scholarships and
awards.* Retrieved from https://www.nphealthcarefoundation.
org/scholarships-awards-fellowships/

Nurses Educational Funds. (2018). *NEF scholarships and funds.*
Retrieved from https://www.n-e-f.org/about/nef-scholarships
.html

Perna, L. W., Wright-Kim, J., & Jiang, N. (2019). *Penn ahead
research brief. Questioning the calculations: Are colleges complying
with federal and ethical mandates for providing students with
estimated costs?* Retrieved from https://repository.upenn.edu/
ahead_papers/4/

ROTC. (n.d.). *Military scholarships for students & enlisted soldiers.* Retrieved from https://www.goarmy.com/rotc/scholarships.html

U.S. News. (n.d.). *Best online master's in nursing programs.* Retrieved from https://www.usnews.com/education/online -education/nursing/rankings

INDEX